S0-BMW-157

Leon Chaitow is a leading practitioner of osteopathy, naturopathy and acupuncture. He teaches widely in the United Kingdom, Europe, Australia and the United States of America, and is a senior lecturer at the University of Westminster, London. He practices at the Hale Clinic, London and is the bestselling author of a wide range of health guides.

Other titles in this series:

Arthritis
Asthma and Hayfever
Diverticulitis
Hiatus Hernia
High Blood Pressure
Skin Problems
Stomach Ulcers
Tinnitus

Thorsons Natural Health

Prostate Problems

Safe alternatives without drugs

LEON CHAITOW

Thorsons
An Imprint of HarperCollinsPublishers

Thorsons

An Imprint of HarperCollins*Publishers*

77–85 Fulham Palace Road,

Hammersmith, London W6 8JB

First published by Thorsons 1988

This revised edition 1998

10 9 8 7 6 5 4 3 2 1

© Leon Chaitow 1988, 1998

Leon Chaitow asserts the moral right to

be identified as the author of this work.

A catalogue record for this book

is available from the British Library

ISBN 0 7225 3561 9

Printed and bound in Great Britain by

Caledonian International Book Manufacturing Ltd, Glasgow

All rights reserved. No part of this publication may be

reproduced, stored in a retrieval system, or transmitted,

in any form or by any means, electronic, mechanical,

photocopying, recording or otherwise, without the prior

permission of the publishers.

Contents

Note to Reader vi

Chapter 1 The Prostate – Its Structure
and Function 1

Chapter 2 Possible Problems of the Prostate 8

Chapter 3 Examination and Massage
of the Prostate 24

Chapter 4 The Role of Nutrients in the
Health of the Prostate 30

Chapter 5 Some Self-help Treatments 36

Chapter 6 Zinc and the Prostate 60

Chapter 7 Fats and Essential Fatty Acids:
Their Effects on the Prostate 69

Chapter 8 Nutrient Therapies for Prostate
Problems 77

Chapter 9 Inflammation of the Prostate:
The Vitamin C Strategy 105

Chapter 10 The Key to Prostate Health 114

Index 136

Note to Reader

While the author of this work has made every effort to ensure that the information contained in this book is as accurate and up to date as possible at the time of publication, medical and pharmaceutical knowledge is constantly changing and the application of it to particular circumstances depends on many factors. Therefore it is recommended that readers always consult a qualified medical specialist for individual advice. This book should not be used as an alternative to seeking specialist medical advice, which should be sought before any action is taken. The author and publishers cannot be held responsible for any errors and omissions that may be found in the text, or any actions that may be taken by the reader as a result of any reliance on the information contained in the text, which is taken entirely at the reader's own risk.

1

The Prostate – Its Structure and Function

For many men the problems which are common with the prostate gland present serious health complications, affecting not only their lives but often the lives of their families too. Medical research has shown that one man in two will develop prostatic hypertrophy (enlargement of the prostate gland) between the ages of 40 and 60. The optimistic view of this rather dismal statistic is that one man in two will *avoid* prostate problems. This implies that prostate problems are not inevitable, not simply a 'part of growing older'. It would also suggest that it might be possible to isolate the reasons for the difference between those men who do and those who do not develop an enlarged prostate, with all its associated difficulties.

We will go on to examine the various types of prostate problems and their concomitant symptoms later in the book, but first it might be helpful to study the structure and function of this important but somewhat mysterious gland.

In the adult man a healthy prostate is about the size and shape of a walnut. It is partly muscular and partly glandular in construction, and is located at the base of the bladder. Its broad upper surface lies just behind the pubic bone, and it narrows in shape to an apex through which the urethra – the tube which drains urine from the bladder – passes along with the ejaculatory ducts. Its major function is to produce a fluid which acts as a carrier for sperm; without this fluid a man would be sterile.

The position of the prostate means that should it become enlarged and consequences can be twofold: first, any swelling squeezes the urethra, causing difficulty in passing urine; second, such enlargement may also restrict the passage of spermatic fluid resulting in problems with fertility. Although this in itself need not result in sexual dysfunction, the bladder problems which are often associated with an enlarged prostate can lead to impotence.

At birth the prostate is largely undeveloped, but by puberty it will have almost doubled in size as the secondary sexual characteristics, such as body and facial hair, and deepening of the voice, occur. During the years up until about the age of 30, there is a continuing development of the glandular aspect of the prostate,

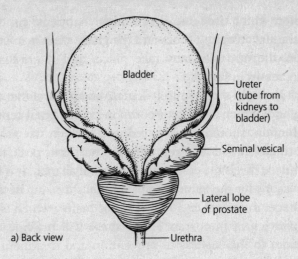

a) Back view

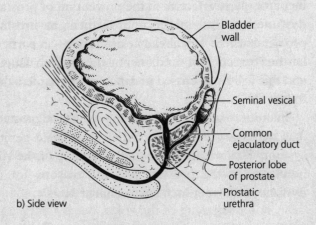

b) Side view

Figure 1 The prostate gland

after which time one of two things happens: either a gradual atrophy occurs and the gland shrinks in size; or, the opposite may take place, and it gradually increases in size.

It would seem entirely logical and natural that the gland, which is a major component of sexual reproduction, should begin to reduce slowly in size as the primary function of reproduction passes its peak, and indeed this is the case in at least half of all men. It is the reasons for the failure of this normal shrinking to take place, in the other 50 per cent of males, which is of paramount importance. For these will provide the clues to the successful prevention and treatment of prostate enlargement. One area that has been shown to be particularly effective in the prevention of prostate dysfunction, and in the improvement of prostate problems where they already exist, is diet – in particular the correction of fundamental dietary imbalances, and this will be discussed in detail in the chapters that follow.

In order to understand fully the role of the prostate, it is necessary to examine briefly the male genital system. This will help our understanding of the vulnerability of the prostate and the reasons for its dysfunction having such far-reaching effects.

The Male Genital System

This comprises the testes (testicles); the vas deferens; the seminal vesicles and the ejaculatory ducts as well as the penis and scrotum. The male germ cell, the spermatozoa, is produced by the reproductive glands, the testes, which hang in the scrotal bag outside the abdominal cavity. This means that the testes are maintained at a temperature which is a degree or two below that of the body as a whole and this is important for sperm production.

The spermatozoa are formed in that part of the testis known as the body. From here they pass into the epididymis, which in turn leads to a muscular sperm duct or the vas deferens. The two ducts (one from each testis) pass through the spermatic cord into the inguinal canal and on into the abdominal cavity. Here the ducts leave the spermatic cord to pass into the pelvis, behind the bladder and into the prostate, where they link with the seminal vesicles (which produce some of the transport fluid for the sperm) to form the ejaculatory duct.

The ejaculatory ducts run through the posterior part of the prostate gland, and finally open into the prostatic urethra.

The secretion produced by the prostate is squeezed into the urethra just prior to ejaculation; here it is mixed with the suspension of spermatozoa and the fluid produced by the seminal vesicles. The final mixture is called seminal fluid and this is what is ejaculated during sexual intercourse.

A healthy prostate allows free micturition (passing of urine) as well as sexual function. To present a programme which maintains this highly desirable state of affairs, and promotes full recovery if problems are already manifest, is the main aim of this book.

Recent research has shown that prostate problems are increasing dramatically. At the turn of the century they were rare and yet now prostate problems are a common complaint in the elderly citizens of the US and Europe. This would imply a direct link between the way of life, and in particular the diet, of twentieth-century man and dysfunction of the prostate and that the solution must therefore lie in a radical alteration of that way of life and diet. It is not by chance that the only animals to suffer in any significant numbers from prostate problems are dogs. The unnatural dietary and general conditions of life of many dogs, reflecting that of their masters, makes this understandable, since these are the very factors which are largely responsible for the condition in man as well.

When the prostate is abnormally enlarged, and causing problems such as those which are discussed in the following chapter, surgery is often the medical answer. Such an approach, however, is in no sense of the word a cure. It simply excises the offending gland, sometimes with less than satisfactory results. The tragedy of this approach has been that it has largely blinded medical science of the possibility of an effective *preventive* approach. Since it is possible simply to remove the gland, why bother to stop it from enlarging in the first place?

This is a very similar story to that associated with tonsils. For many years these were removed surgically almost as soon as they became a problem. Nowadays of course the folly of such an approach has been driven home by the indisputable evidence that such operations lead to a greatly decreased resistance to infection. Tonsils are only removed now as a last resort.

Yet tonsils were always amenable to a dietary approach which detoxified the body and so reduced the work load placed on these filtration organs. In a similar manner the prostate is amenable to a nutritional approach, which provides it with essential nutrients. It is a deficiency in such essential nutrients that is the major precursor of prostate enlargement. This means that there are effective measures that any individual can take to ensure a great deal of protection from the danger of an enlarged prostate. There are also effective treatments which can be used to reduce the troublesome symptoms of a prostate if it has already enlarged, without resorting to surgery. Once we have established the types of problem to which the prostate is prone we will move on to an investigation of these methods.

2
Possible Problems of the Prostate

There are two major forms of prostate problem which experience has shown are responsive to self-help measures: first, prostatitis, an inflammation and usually infection of the prostate gland; and second, hypertrophy of the prostate, where the gland enlarges, resulting in a variety of unpleasant symptoms which we will discuss below. The enlargement of the prostate is also known, more accurately, as benign prostatic hypertrophy (BPH); this is the term which we will use henceforth.

Prostate Cancer

There is of course a third possible disease of the prostate, cancer of that organ, but this is not within the scope of a self-help book. Cancer of the prostate is the major form of cancer affecting the reproductive system of males. Preventive measures (outlined in later chapters) will almost certainly stop the gland degenerating from simple enlargement to a state of malignancy. Such a progression is by no means inevitable, although malignancy seldom occurs unless the gland has displayed enlargement (BPH) previously.

When the prostate is being checked for possible malignancy a number of methods are used, including direct palpation via the rectum (*see Chapter 3*), ultrasound employed rectally, measurement of prostate-specific antigens (PSA) in the bloodstream, and scan technology methods.

There is a great deal of anecdotal evidence to support the use of the measures suggested in this book as a complementary (but not alternative) approach to treatment of prostatic cancer, which is increasingly likely to be successfully treated as modern methods have evolved.

Complementary approaches to treatment of prostate cancer should not be purely self-selected and self-applied if this condition has been diagnosed, but should be followed under the supervision of a suitably qualified and licensed health care professional.

Acute Prostatitis

In some cases acute prostatitis is the result of a sexually transmitted agent, such as venereal disease. This is, however, not the major cause of prostatitis, which usually derives from an infection in some other part of the body. The presenting symptoms are usually a combination of fever (38.9°C/102°F) and flu-like aches, together with shivering. This is accompanied by aching in the back and between the legs, with major discomfort felt on sitting. There will also be a great deal of discomfort or even pain on passing water and during bowel movements.

Some experts believe that, in certain cases, excessive sexual activity (including masturbation) depletes the prostate of zinc (sperm has a very high zinc content) which acts partially to protect the region from infection. In other words, infection and therefore inflammation may be the result of the environment being made more amenable for invading microorganisms, whether these be bacteria or yeasts.

Medical treatment of prostatitis usually involves bedrest and a course of antibiotics for about 10 days with copious amounts of liquid, followed by a further week or so of rest. During the entire course of treatment no alcohol or sexual activity is allowed. Recurrence of the problem is common if the rules of rest and diet are not followed – or if the underlying causes are not dealt with.

Chronic Prostatitis and Infection
(Bacterial or Yeast)

There is also a chronic form of prostatitis, triggered usually by a persistent infection of some part of the body such as the bowels, teeth or the tonsils. This produces recurring attacks of slight fever, sexual difficulties and an ache in the low back as well as between the legs and in the back passage. Medical treatment usually involves a course of sulpha drugs and massage of the prostate.

There is a close relationship between bladder infection and prostatitis as well as urethritis, an inflammation of the urethra. These infections may relate to bacteria or to overgrowth of the yeast *Candida albicans*. It is often difficult to distinguish between prostate, bladder or urethral infections as they often coexist, despite the fact that prostatic fluid contains an antibacterial factor which inhibits some forms of infection (which may account for the fact that men suffer from fewer urinary infections than women). Ways to help to identify the possibility of prostate inflammation being caused by yeast overgrowth is given below – and suggested treatment methods will be found in Chapter 9.

Heavy Metal and Pesticide Toxicity

Another major cause of chronic prostatitis (and BPH) has been identified as exposure to, and absorption of, chemical compounds such as pesticides as well as toxic heavy metals, most particularly cadmium, which has been found in concentrated levels in that organ in many patients with enlargement of the prostate.

Yeast Overgrowth

The use of antibiotics and/or steroid medication (cortisone, for example) can lead to the spread in the intestinal tract and the body generally of yeasts which are normally controlled by 'friendly' bacteria (which live in our intestinal tracts, performing essential tasks including yeast control); these bacteria are damaged by such medication. The main yeast engaged in such activity is Candida albicans, best known for causing thrush (mainly in women but commonly in men as well).

Candida is dangerous because of its ability to turn from a simple yeast into an aggressive mycelial fungus which puts down 'rootlets' (rhizomes) into the mucous membrane of the intestinal tract, so permitting undesirable toxins to move from the gut into the bloodstream, with the strong possibility of allergic and toxic reactions taking place.

Among the many symptoms which have been catalogued in people affected in this way are a range of digestive symptoms (bloating, swings from diarrhoea to constipation and back), chronic urinary tract infections, fatigue, muscle aches, emotional disturbances, 'foggy' brain symptoms and skin problems (as well as menstrual problems in women). The frequency with which such symptoms are suffered by the general population is enormous.

Laboratory tests to 'prove' yeast involvement are commonly inaccurate, mainly because almost everyone on the planet has some yeast living in their digestive tract – simply finding it there does not help to determine just how widespread its presence is.

Diagnosis by symptoms is more accurate; if an anti-Candida programme makes the symptoms vanish or improve greatly, this confirms the diagnosis.

One of the most useful tests involves a sugar-loading test – a sample of blood is taken, then 100 g of sugar are consumed on an empty stomach, then another blood sample is taken one hour later. This test assesses the level of alcohol in the blood before and after the sugar intake, because yeast – and some bacteria – can turn sugar into alcohol rapidly in the intestines.

When to Suspect Candida

Candida overgrowth may prove to be a factor in your health problems if after examining the lists below you find that one item or more from each applies to you.

a Have you:
a history of long-term antibiotic usage (one long period of taking them – more than two months – or more than four courses in any one year)? This would have damaged the normal flora and allowed the always present yeast to spread.
ever taken a course of tetracycline (or any other antibiotic) to treat acne for more than one month?

b And, do you (or have you):
suffered from persistent prostatitis or cystitis (bladder infection) or urethritis?
had ringworm or athlete's foot?
had cravings for sugar or bread or alcohol?

c And are you currently suffering from:
fatigue?
digestive bloating or 'irritable bowel'?
'foggy brain' (short-term memory difficulties, concentration problems)?
widespread muscular aches and pains?
thrush?
loss of sexual interest?

If you consider that you may have a Candida overgrowth, or if this has been diagnosed by a responsible health care professional, you may wish to consult an expert who deals with such problems, or to read more about it (see my book *Candida Albicans – Could Yeast Be Your Problem?*, Thorsons, 1995).

The detailed recommendations given in Chapter 8 represent an absolute minimum anti-Candida strategy which should be carried out for not less than three months. Ideally this should be under the supervision of a suitably trained nutritional expert (naturopath, medical herbalist, clinical ecologist, nutritional counsellor, dietitian, etc.). Conditions associated with fungal infection, whether these involve the skin, the intestinal tract or the urinary tract, may appear to be worse for the first few weeks of an anti-Candida diet (*see Chapter 8*).

Symptoms

Prostatitis may occur at any age, although it is more common in later years as the chances of BPH increase. Thus it can be seen that one of the precursors of an inflamed prostate is an enlarged one, although there are other possible causes.

In older men the presenting symptoms of prostatitis may not involve any fever, but may simply be a degree of urgency in wanting to pass water, with an accompanying hesitancy or difficulty in controlling the flow.

In such cases bacteria are usually found to be present on culture of the urine (*see notes on cranberry juice or extracts in Chapter 8*).

Other men may present with symptoms such as frequency of urination, difficulty in urination and foul-smelling urine as well as cramp-like sensations in the loins, etc.

In many cases the only symptoms of an inflamed prostate are vague sensations of discomfort in the lower back and mild difficulty on urination.

Self-help for Prostatitis

There are a number of self-help methods which have proved extremely effective in the treatment of prostatitis, including detoxification diets, dealing with food or environmental allergies, or treatment of yeast infections which may, as mentioned, be a major cause of the problem. Supplementation of specific nutrients such as vitamin C (in very high doses), essential fatty acids (such as are found in cold-pressed flaxseed oil, for example) and zinc may be called for.

These and other self-help methods are dealt with fully in the chapters that follow.

Benign Prostatic Hypertrophy (BPH)

About 60 per cent of men between the ages of 40 and 60 have a prostate gland which has enlarged.

Prostate conditions are a major health problem throughout the developed countries. Yet such conditions are hardly known in the underdeveloped world. This can only lead to the conclusion that the causes of such conditions lie in the diet or lifestyle of industrialized man.

The actual increase in size of the prostate causes an interference with the urethra and the opening of the bladder to this urinary channel.

Some experts believe that as men grow older the conversion of the male hormone testosterone (produced in the testicles and the adrenal glands) to a more active form – dihydrotestosterone – is accelerated, leading to more rapid growth of tissues in the prostate and to the problems this causes.

The reasons for this increase in dihydrotestosterone seems to be a combination of several factors – including a deficiency in specific enzymes which normally control the levels of conversion of testosterone to its more active form. This deficiency, it is thought, may be due to increased levels, in older men, of the female hormone oestrogen, and to increased levels of another hormone, prolactin, which causes the prostate to absorb more testosterone – which turns into the growth-promoting dihydrotestosterone and enlarges the prostate. Prolactin is stimulated by the consumption of alcohol (beer in particular) and by stress. These effects can be helped by selective nutrient supplementation (zinc and vitamin B_6), as will be explained in Chapter 8.

High levels of chemicals such as dioxin and others common in pesticides (and other environmental contaminants) help to stimulate the levels of dihydrotestosterone in the prostate gland. There are a number of nutritional tactics which can assist in the elimination of these, as will be outlined in later chapters.

The first indication of a growth in the size of the prostate is usually a painless increase in the frequency of urination. A man will suddenly find that he has to pass water, often at about 2 or 3 a.m. at night. Eventually this need will become more urgent and more frequent, affecting both day and night, until other symptoms are noted, such as difficulty in commencing urination.

Any attempt at straining is useless and can have a further detrimental effect by increasing the pressure in the lower abdomen, so reducing the flow even more. Once urination has commenced, control of the noticeably weaker urine stream may become difficult, ending in a dribble which may take some time to stop.

There may or may not be sexual difficulties associated with prostate hypertrophy, although usually such difficulties are connected with associated infection or other accompanying conditions.

The enlarged prostate may be pressing on the urethra, restricting the flow of urine and making control of urination difficult. If the enlargement is marked it may result in the prostate blocking the opening of the bladder into the urethra, thus obstructing the flow of urine completely. The more effort exerted, the more blocked the passage of urine becomes.

It is possible for the strength of the peak stream of urine to be tested medically. This test should be conducted:

- if the need to urinate increases in frequency to more than five times in 24 hours;
- if you experience sudden, abrupt stopping of the urine flow during urination;
- if there is an obvious weakening of the force of the flow of urine;
- if the stream of urine becomes noticeably thinner;
- or if you feel any pain, or pass any blood, during urination.

Always seek medical advice if any of these symptoms present, and it is imperative to embark on self-help measures if deterioration is to be avoided and improvement achieved.

Apart from any other consideration, a reduced flow of urine may result in a small amount of urine being left in the bladder, giving rise to infection which could even result in damage to the kidneys. Thus it is very important that problems concerned with urination are resolved.

Various problems will result in a reduced urine flow rate, including narrowing of the urethra from an old infection; stones in the kidneys; tumours in the bladder or elsewhere, or the consequences of neurological damage to the area. However, the most likely cause in middle-aged men is BPH.

Other Symptoms and their Implications

As well as the alteration to the urine flow, there may well be the development of associated symptoms, such as pain in the lower abdomen or between the legs, in the back or, as in sciatica, in the legs only.

The strength of the symptoms varies from person to person; in some they may be slight, in others very marked. If such associated symptoms arise over a period of weeks, rather than months, then medical advice should be sought as the problem may involve more than simple enlargement of the prostate (BPH), which is usually pain- and symptom-free, apart from the urinary difficulties already discussed.

Note

It should be clear that the advice given in this book relating to BPH is not intended to be used in cases of prostate cancer. BPH stands for benign prostate hypertrophy – the word *benign* indicates that the enlargement (hypertrophy) of the gland is not malignant. Check your symptoms against the summary below and answer the questionnaire on page 22. If in any doubt, consult your doctor.

Summary of Symptoms of BPH

- progressive urinary frequency
- urgency, especially at night
- hesitancy and lack of control of passage of urine
- difficulty in cessation of passage of urine (dribbling)
- reduced force of urine stream
- enlarged, non-tender, non-lumpy prostate
- possible presence of blood in the urine if obstruction is prolonged
- possible associated infection of the bladder due to stagnant urine.

Prostate Self-Assessment Questionnaire

Answer as follows:

- a *yes* means this is almost always so
- a *sometimes* means that this is the case once a week or more, but not constantly
- *rarely* means less than weekly.
- if a question does not apply to you at all, do not answer it.
- Score 3 points for a *yes* answer.
- Score 2 points for a *sometimes* answer.
- Score 1 point for a *rarely* answer.
- a *no* answer (question 5 only) scores 0 points.

Q1. Do you have difficulty in urinating, whether it's starting the flow or stopping it (i.e. a dribble continuing for some time), or find that you notice a burning sensation when passing urine?
yes/sometimes/rarely

Q2. Do you have to get up at night to pass water?
yes/sometimes/rarely

Q3. If you answered yes to either Q1 or Q2, do you feel any discomfort in the lower back, loins or back of the legs when urinating?
yes/sometimes/rarely

Q4. Have you noticed a diminishment, or loss, of sexual drive?
yes/sometimes/rarely

Q5. Have you been told by your doctor that you have a prostate enlargement?
yes/no

Scoring

- 0 to 2 indicates no real problem.
- 3 to 5 indicates a problem and that the advice in this book should be heeded. A checkup or examination would also be recommended if improvement is not noted within a month or so of introducing the nutritional (zinc supplementation, etc.) programme as outlined later in the book.

- A score above 5 indicates prostate dysfunction and calls for an immediate medical examination. Start the self-help programme straightaway in conjunction with your medical advice.

This self-assessment is not meant to take the place of responsible advice from a health-care practitioner, but as a guide to your possible current state of prostate enlargement. It may be repeated from time to time (at not less than monthly intervals) in order to aid in assessing your progress as the self-help programme is underway.

We will next consider a method of examination of the prostate by direct finger contact. This is *not a self-administered* examination, but requires a co-operative and gentle friend or family member. It is not essential but is useful, both for keeping a check on progress during self-treatment, and as an actual form of treatment by prostate massage.

3

Examination and Massage of the Prostate

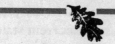

It is standard practice for a doctor to check the health of the prostate gland by feeling its contours and texture during a medical examination. This is known as palpation. There is nothing to prevent such an examination being done by a friend or member of the family, in order to provide guidance as to the degree of hardness, enlargement and subsequent improvement, in the gland. Examination and/or massage of the prostate involves the gentle insertion of a gloved finger into the rectum, in a precise manner, and this obviously calls for a degree of mutual trust and respect.

The Normal Prostate

The normal gland is about the size of a walnut with two lobes (as in a shelled walnut) and a central groove. It should therefore feel about 2.5 to 3cm in length, with a shallow groove in the midline. The correct consistency has been described as the texture you feel if you make a tight fist, and then with the other hand feel the muscular tissue which lies between the base of the thumb and the base of the index finger (*see Figure 2*). This is a muscular but not rock hard texture; neither is it soft and mushy.

Examining the Prostate Manually

It is best if the person to be examined empties his bladder and bowels before the examination starts (although it is still likely that an urge to pass urine will be felt during the examination). Then he should kneel on the floor before a low bed and rest his chest and abdomen on the bed so that he is quite comfortable and relaxed.

An alternative position is for the person being examined to lie on the bed, facing the edge, with his knees tucked up to his chest. The examiner then stands in front of the person and, by leaning over his pelvic area, can carry out the examination.

The examiner should wear surgical gloves (most chemists sell these) and lubricate the index finger – the

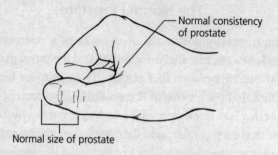

Figure 2 Guide to checking size and consistency
of the prostate gland

examining one – with a sterile gel such as Vaseline or
K-Y. Never use anything to lubricate which is medi-
cated or perfumed. Check that the nail on the examining finger is well trimmed to avoid the possibility of
scratching or causing unnecessary discomfort.

The examiner should then press the examining finger gently against the person's anus. At first no effort
should be made to penetrate the rectum. As the external muscles relax, he should insert the finger, gently
but firmly, to its limit. If any resistance is felt, no force
should be used, but wait for the muscles to relax. Once
the examiner has penetrated the rectum, he should
press downwards lightly with the pad of the finger tip
and it should be possible to feel a walnut-sized mass;
this is the prostate gland.

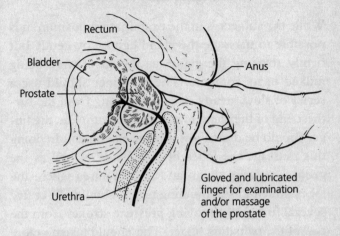

Rectum

Bladder

Prostate

Anus

Gloved and lubricated
finger for examination
and/or massage
of the prostate

Urethra

Figure 3 Manual examination of the prostate

If the length of the gland does not seem excessive, no more than 3cm, say, then it is probably not enlarged or only very slightly so. In some cases it can reach the size of an orange. It should feel smooth and firm to the examining finger, not soft and mushy, or hard and nodular. The examiner should be able to detect the midline groove. If the prostate feels lumpy (nodular) and very hard, then medical advice should be sought.

Massaging the Prostate

While the subject is in the examination position, it is possible to massage the gland lightly, by gently but firmly stroking the gland, as though it were being milked of its contents. The examiner should use a series of slow, steady strokes, working from the furthest end of the gland towards the rectum (i.e. the finger should be drawn towards the examiner). In doing this massage the lobes of the gland, as well as the groove between them, and also the area where the lobes attach to surrounding tissue, should all receive several firm, slow-moving pressure strokes from the pad of the palpating finger. This should take no more than a minute. Such massaging can greatly assist in normalizing a congested gland, especially when combined with the dietary and other methods to be discussed later.

During the massage there may well be a desire to pass urine which may become uncontrollable. Suitable precautions should therefore be taken before the massage starts, such as placing disposable absorbent material underneath the subject.

If the prostate palpates as nodular or lumpy, then it should not be massaged. Nor should it be massaged if it is very soft and slushy. Only perform the massage if the gland feels firm and not lumpy, but enlarged beyond the size of a walnut.

The massage can be done once or twice a week during the treatment phase, and examination can be carried out once a fortnight or so to assess the improvement which will usually be noted as the gland slowly returns to a normal size.

Subsequent to massage of the prostate there may be noted a distinct improvement in the control of passing of urine. This may be only temporary at first, but if the dietary and other methods outlined in the first chapter are also being used, this should steadily become permanent.

4

The Role of Nutrients in the Health of the Prostate

In this chapter we will take a general look at some of the nutrients which are vital in the safe self-help treatment and, of course, in the prevention of prostate problems. Later in the book we examine in detail the evidence for their value, as well as providing information as to sources and amounts required. But for now, we present an outline of the sorts of nutrients and the ways in which these are known to affect underlying biochemical changes.

It is sometimes believed that as there are so many different nutrients which are useful in dealing with the prostate, any one of these is adequate to the task of normalizing the gland. However, the fact is that there are a number of vital nutrients which should be used together in the diet, taken either in food, the ideal way, or as supplements, the practical manner of ensuring an adequate intake.

The prostate gland is a very complex organ and its function involves a variety of factors interacting in a carefully balanced system. The changes which are involved in BPH represent an imbalance in this network which is related to the presence of, and interaction between, male hormones such as testosterone, and other hormones and substances such as prolactin, oestradiol, etc.

The first named of these, testosterone, decreases in its presence in the body from the age of about 40, whereas the others increase at this time. The ultimate effect of these changes in older men is often to increase the presence in the prostate of a derivative of testosterone called dihydrotestosterone (DHT). Normally DHT is excreted from the gland in sufficient quantities to prevent enlargement occurring and to maintain the prostate at its normal size. However, if there should be an imbalance between the hormones, and this is common in later life, DHT is not adequately excreted, causing the prostate to swell. When an enlarged prostate is examined it is possible to detect three or four times the normal levels of DHT.

Nutrients such as the mineral zinc as well as a high protein intake have been shown to reduce the levels of, or the activity of, an enzyme which aids in the conversion of testosterone to DHT. This enzyme is known as 5-alpha reductase, and its activity increases (making prostate enlargement more likely) when the diet is high in carbohydrates and low in protein. Its activity is reduced (thus decreasing the likelihood of prostate enlargement) when the diet is high in protein and low in carbohydrate. Similarly, when zinc levels are high the activity of 5-alpha reductase is lowered, thus reducing the chance of prostate enlargement occurring. Unfortunately, zinc levels in modern man are seldom adequate, and so with this deficiency comes an increase in 5-alpha reductase levels, leading to high levels of the testosterone derivative DHT, and so an enlargement of the prostate. (We will be looking at the best ways of achieving zinc adequacy later.) Zinc has a further role in helping the prostate, since it reduces the secretion of the substance prolactin, thereby increasing testosterone uptake by the prostate.

It has been shown that individuals with BPH also have an imbalance in the quantities of, and ratios between, certain substances called essential fatty acids (EFAs). There are a number of these extremely important nutrient factors (for details of sources, see pp. 75), but basically they can be divided into three groups: linoleic acid, linolenic acid, and arachidonic acid. Correction of a deficiency in these, by nutritional alterations and supplementation, has been shown to improve dramatically the condition of individuals with BPH. (Results of trials involving this strategy will be given when EFAs are discussed in more detail; see pp. 73.

The building blocks of protein are called amino acids, and there are over 20 of these. As mentioned previously, the use of a high-protein diet can be helpful in normalizing the prostate (although there are other good reasons why a very high-protein diet is not desirable long-term for many people). It has been found that three of the amino acids taken in combination – glycine, alinine, and glutamic acid – are capable of dramatically improving BPH, and we will examine evidence of this, as well as the dosages recommended, in the chapters that follow.

One of the greatest dangers accompanying BPH is that of a possible malignant change occurring. It has been noted that the breakdown products of cholesterol are cancer-producing, and that these have a tendency to accumulate in the prostate gland when enlarged. For this reason, as well as for general health improvement, it is important for cholesterol levels to be maintained at safe limits. What these limits are and how to achieve them as discussed in a later chapter, but they do involve a reduction in sugar intake as well as ensuring an adequate fibre intake. There are other good reasons for a dietary pattern which includes a high fibre content, not the least being the need for bowel regularity. It has been shown that constipation is a frequent co-symptom with BPH and there is every chance that the long-term increase in pressure caused by constipation, as well as the tendency this produces for straining, are factors in the production of congestion in the lower pelvic region in which the prostate lies. Improvement in bowel function, through correct dietary practices, must be an element in any prostate self-help programme.

These, in brief, are the nutrient strategies which are necessary for coping with existing prostate enlargement, as well as for preventing its occurrence in the first place. No one of these elements alone is sufficient; rather it is necessary to restructure the diet to provide adequate levels of protein, limit refined carbohydrate intake and ensure that zinc and its co-factors are adequately present, along with a correct quantity and balance of essential fatty acids. Specific amino acid combinations should also be added, and control exercised to maintain healthy cholesterol levels. All these should be combined with sufficient fibre intake to ensure a sound bowel function.

This may sound complicated, but fortunately the different components of this approach to correct an enlarged prostate interact, and so a basic dietary approach will take care of most of the requirements.

There are other elements which may be incorporated into a prostate gland health programme, including extracts of pollen, which are noted as being helpful, as well as the use of ginseng and extracts of the fruit of the palm tree, Sereno Repens. These will be outlined briefly in subsequent chapters as adding to the overall value of the nutritional approach.

It is important that the programme presented in later chapters is followed in full, not just in part. There would doubtless be benefit derived from taking just one element, such as zinc, and hoping for an improvement. However, the various elements of the diet should be seen as interacting, and all should be used to achieve the greatest long-term benefit.

5
Some Self-help Prostate Treatments

Body Mechanics and the Prostate

Structure and function are obviously interrelated and mutually interdependent. The way something is constructed determines the use to which it can be put (try cutting bread with a toothbrush); similarly, the way something is used will alter its structure (even a sharp knife becomes dull with regular use). The human body is constructed to be used in a set number of ways. Used incorrectly, the body's shape and structure can be altered. For instance, posture can vary and alter with occupation and habitual use, and as the structure (posture) alters, the function of the component parts is forced to alter too.

Take someone who is habitually stooped: their chest cage will be depressed rather than open, and their abdominal contents, the organs and structures of the digestive and reproductive systems, will be crowded. This produces alterations in the way these organs function, as well as increasing the degree of congestion in them.

In good body mechanics the chest is held high, the diaphragm (which separates the chest from the abdominal cavity) is also high, and the abdominal wall is flat and firm. When posture is poor and mechanics inferior, the chest is depressed, the diaphragm is unable to move adequately up and down with respiration, and the abdominal wall bulges out as the contents of the abdominal cavity are pushed down towards the floor of the pelvis. This creates problems not just in the pelvic region and the prostate, of course; it can also cause the liver and stomach to alter their positions, as well as crowding of the intestinal canal. Functional changes take place in these regions as a consequence, and are often responsible for health problems, some of which can be quite serious. The drag of the organs on their supporting ligaments, for instance, can produce strains and tears such as occur in hiatus hernia, etc. The circulation of blood to, and through, these regions is dramatically altered in such a situation. The only source of drainage of blood, lymph, etc., from the pelvic organs is via the abdominal veins, which are severely affected by distention of the abdominal contents forwards or downwards.

These factors are thought by many eminent researchers to relate to the problems of bladder and prostate experienced by so many men, and to the malposition of the uterus in women, which can lead to period problems and pregnancy difficulties.

The nerve supply to these organs is also dependent upon sound body mechanics, involving the lower back and pelvic structures. Thus postural factors and the way the body is used are of importance in our assessment of the causes of prostate dysfunction. Sagging abdominal contents, poorly functioning diaphragmatic movement in breathing, long periods of stasis when sitting, inadequate exercise and, as mentioned above, straining at stool usually linked to constipation, all add to the problems of the region in terms of poor circulation, poor nerve supply and poor drainage.

Congestion leads to altered nutritional status of the region, for no matter how good the diet, if the nutrients cannot adequately be transported and the waste products adequately drained, the end result is an impoverished region with the potential for disease and poor function. This is the pattern in prostate hypertrophy in many men.

What Can Be Done about Such Postural Habits?

Bodywork such as is offered by osteopaths, chiropractors, physiotherapists and massage therapists can offer the opportunity for normalizing shortened and restricted soft tissues as well as loosening up joint restrictions – which are necessary precursors to postural re-education such as is taught by Alexander Technique experts or yoga instructors. Exercises which stretch and rehabilitate abnormal function (such as breathing, which is of major importance) are also useful adjuncts to normalization of the mechanics of the body. Some exercises are suggested in this chapter, but nothing can take the place of expert advice and instruction.

Sexual Factors

When a man has intercourse, the following sequence of events occurs in the region of the prostate: initial stimulation, followed by erection, increase the prostate's secretion of fluids; with orgasm the seminal vesicles and the vas deferens contract, as do the ejaculatory ducts, and the sperm is delivered through the urethra; this is followed by relaxation of tension and dissipation of congestion in the region.

Sexual stimulation which is not followed by orgasm has many potentially deleterious effects, including inflammation of the urethra, local discomfort in the perineal area due to congestion, as well as possible impotence and, as would be expected, prostate enlargement accompanying the chronic congestion resulting from this practice. In short, sexual practices culminating in orgasm are not damaging to a man's health, but interruption of the cycle leading to orgasm can be.

In general terms, then, the normalization of posture and regular exercise are to be encouraged. This may involve advice and/or treatment from a suitably qualified practitioner, such as an osteopath, to correct any faults in spinal and pelvic mechanics. Also, it is essential to avoid any straining over bowel movements, and to this end the dietary advice to be found later in this book will be of great assistance. In addition, by using this knowledge of the link between structure and function, a number of effective self-treatments can be devised.

Hydrotherapy

Forms of water therapy (hydrotherapy) can be extremely effective in reducing local congestion of the pelvic floor. There are two methods of hydrotherapy advocated in cases of hypertrophy of the prostate, as well as several general 'constitutional' (i.e. whole-body) methods which assist in circulatory enhancement, which indirectly helps the prostate.

Method I: Prostate Specific
The first method involves local irrigation using a cool saline solution. This is not an enema in the sense of attempting to enhance elimination via the bowel.

Rather it is a means of applying a cold liquid to a congested area in order to stimulate drainage.

An enema bag, containing about 1 litre of water into which 2 teaspoons of salt have been dissolved, is required. The temperature of the water should have been reduced to about 13° to 15°C (55° to 60°F), by refrigeration. (Mix the salt with the water, add to the bag and refrigerate until used.)

Bedtime is a good time to perform the local irrigation. The bowels should have been opened some time previously, so that the need for defecation is not current. Sitting upright on the toilet, the patient introduces the tip of the application tube into the rectum, using a little lubricant on the tip for ease of entry. The enema bag containing the water should be suitably suspended nearby. It must of course be higher than the body of the individual, so that gravity will allow the water to enter the rectum with ease.

The initial amount allowed into the rectum is about 100 ml (4 fl oz/approximately ½ a cup) of cold saline mixture. This is retained for about half a minute and then allowed to be expelled into the toilet bowl. This is followed, after a minute or so of rest, by the same procedure. Altogether the pattern is repeated seven or eight times, which should use up the whole litre of water.

The method described produces an alternating hot and cold effect locally, within the rectum, and this closely approximates the prostate circulatory system. The cold applications cool the area down, and natural body heat warms it up again during the rest period between irrigations.

This should be done three times weekly by anyone with BPH. Benefits will soon be noted and the practice may be reduced in frequency as improvement continues.

Method 2: Prostate Specific

A further measure which may be useful is the alternating immersion of the pelvis in hot and cold water. This is valuable because it not only gives relief to painful and distressing symptoms, but also helps to reduce congestion and thus to restore normal structure. It is especially helpful in relieving what is known as connective tissue stasis, an extreme congestion of the tissues, and is in this way a unique therapeutic agent.

Run about 12 cm of hot water (not hot enough to scald but as hot as is tolerable) in the bath and sit in this for a half to one minute. Alongside the bath should be a bowl sufficiently deep to allow for some 12 cm of cold water, and large enough to sit in – a large plastic bowl or an old-fashioned hip bath would do. (Years ago a proper portable bath was made for this purpose, which had a sloping back and a sitting arrangement so that the feet could rest comfortably on the floor whilst the pelvis was immersed.)

The idea of the bath is to sit, with the knees bent, so that the buttocks and the pelvic area (up to no higher than the navel) are covered with water. After the immersion in hot water, transfer rapidly to the cold water for a further half to one minute, after which the pattern may be repeated once more, of hot followed by cold, for the same lengths of time.

If it is not possible to arrange a second bath or bowl for the cold immersion, then the water from the hot bath should be drained away and replaced with cold water. This delays the contrast element of the procedure somewhat, but is better than nothing.

Between immersions keep up the level of warmth by wrapping yourself in a towel, at the same time ensuring that the room itself is warm.

This alternation of hot and cold has a most beneficial effect on local circulation and may be performed daily if possible, or on alternate days, when the irrigation (Method 1) is not being used.

If it is not possible to alternate immersion in hot and cold water, hot and cold towels may be used instead to create a similar effect. For this a series of towels is wrung out in hot water and placed over the lower groin and lower back, and between the legs, ensuring the anus is well-covered. Repeated reapplications of hot towels to these regions are carried out over a 15- to 20-minute period. The heat should be strong, but obviously not excessive enough to cause any discomfort in this sensitive region.

Each towel should remain in position for a minute or two, before being replaced. After about 15 minutes a cold application should be made in the same areas by wringing out towels in cold water, applying them quickly and leaving them in place for a minute or so.

Method 3: Constitutional Hydrotherapy for Circulatory Enhancement

The results of important hydrotherapy research in London involving 100 volunteers were published in *The European* on 22nd and 29th April, 1993.

The Thrombosis Research Institute (which conducted the research) claims that the use of this form of self-treatment proves without question the dramatic value of carefully graduated cold baths, regularly taken (six months' daily use is suggested for optimal results).

The Institute, under its director Dr Vijay Kakkar, have now gathered 5,000 volunteers for the next stage of this research into the benefits of what has been called Thermo Regulatory Hydrotherapy (TRH).

The results of the first study showed that when applied correctly the effect of TRH was:

- a boost to sex hormone production which helps regulate both potency in men and fertility in women
- renewed energy: many sufferers from chronic fatigue syndrome were found to improve dramatically

- improved circulation in people with cold
  extremities. Circulation is found to improve rapidly
  with TRH, along with levels of specific enzymes
  which help circulation. This is particularly
  important in prostate hypertrophy, where
  circulation in the pelvic area is likely to be sluggish.
- reduced chances of heart attack and stroke because
  of improved blood-clotting function
- increased levels of white blood cells
- reduced levels of unpleasant menopausal
  symptoms.

The Method of TRH

There are four stages to TRH and it is essential to
'train' the body towards the beneficial response by
going through each of these stages in turn.

- Equipment needed: a bath, a bath thermometer,
  a watch and a bath mat
- The bathroom needs to be at a reasonably
  comfortable temperature – not too cold and not
  very hot.
- The temperature of the water should eventually be
  as it comes from the tap – cold – however it is
  possible to train towards the cold bath by first
  having a tepid bath for a few weeks, gradually
  making the water colder so that it goes below body

heat, until having a really cold bath is no longer
a shock.

- The timing described below can also be modified
so that at first the whole process takes just a few
minutes as the various stages of immersion are
passed through, with a slow increase in the timing
of each stage as well as a reduction in temperature.

Note

When cold water treatments are used in people with
chronic health problems, the degree of stimulus used
(how cold the water is, and how long a time is spent
immersed) needs to be modified so that a very SLOW
increment in contrast is achieved, gradually training
and 'hardening' the body to what is potentially a stress
factor. The TRH programme runs for 80 days, with
the degree of coldness and the length of time in the
water increased only gradually.

To plunge someone who is extremely fragile in their
ability to handle stress of any sort into cold water
straight from the tap would be foolhardy, whereas
taking a shower or bath in 'neutral' (body heat) water
for a week before – extremely gradually – starting
the process of, day by day, getting the water cooler
and cooler, perhaps over a period of months before
tap-cold water is used, is both sensible and effective.

Stage 1

Stand in the bath in cold water (the range recommended is between 12.7° and 18.3°C [59° and 65°F], but
take account of the Note above as to how cold the
water should be in relation to the degree of the subject's fragility/robustness) for between 1 and 5 minutes
once fully used to the process, perhaps after some
weeks, as the internal thermostat (in the hypothalamus
portion of the brain) responds.

Have a non-slip mat in place and avoid standing still
but 'walk' up and down the bath or march on the spot.

Stage 2

When fully used to the standing in cold water process,
perhaps after some weeks, the internal thermostat is
now primed. At this stage after standing for several
minutes, sit in the cold water for another 1 to 5 minutes (ideally the water should be up to the waist – so
that the pooled blood in the lower half of the body is
cooled, further influencing the hypothalamus and
helping to decongest the pelvis).

Stage 3

After another two or three weeks when the daily immersion involves first standing, then sitting, we come to the
most important part of the programme, in which it is
necessary to immerse the entire body up to the neck and
back of the head in cold water. After first standing, then

sitting, lie down in the water so that just the face and head are clear. Gently and slowly move the arms and legs to ensure that the slightly warmer water touching the skin is not static, and the cooling effect continues. This stage ultimately lasts between 10 and 20 minutes, but could be for as little as two minutes at first, with the degree of coldness being adjusted according to sensitivity.

Stage 4

This is for 'rewarming'. Get out of the bath, towel dry and move around for a few minutes. As warming takes place a pleasant glowing sensation will be felt in various precise locations such as the chest, feet, and between the shoulder blades.

The whole sequence, modified by reducing the time and temperature at first, needs to be done daily if the 'training' or 'hardening' effect is to be achieved. Some people find that several cold baths daily improve their function and energy.

Contraindications

This cold water bath method is not recommended for people with well-established heart disease, high blood pressure or chronic diseases who require regular prescription medication – unless a doctor has been consulted as to the use of TRH.

Studies in Germany have shown that repetitive daily cold showers produce, over a three- to six-month period, a marked immune system enhancement with far fewer infections, and with the duration of those infections that do occur (colds/flu) far shorter than in people having hot or warm showers.

Method 4: Constitutional Hydrotherapy – Whole-body Circulation Enhancement

Another approach to 'whole-body' circulation enhancement which has beneficial effects on the prostate is called simply Constitutional Hydrotherapy and was devised by American Naturopaths earlier in the twentieth century as a method of health enhancement. This cannot be self-applied and requires someone to assist. The whole procedure takes around 25 minutes and should be conducted three times a week for at least a month to achieve benefits. It can be undertaken more frequently without harm (there are no risks or contraindications) and can be performed indefinitely as long as benefits are felt.

Constitutional Hydrotherapy (CH) – Home Application
Effects: CH has a non-specific 'balancing' effect, reducing chronic pain, enhancing immune function, boosting circulatory efficiency (which helps the prostate) and promoting healing. There are no contraindications since the degree of temperature contrast in its application can be modified to take account of any degree of

sensitivity, frailty, etc.

Materials:

somewhere to lie down

a full-sized sheet folded in two, or two single sheets

1 blanket (wool if possible)

2 bath towels (when folded in two, each should be able
to reach side to side and from shoulders to hips)

2 hand towels (each should as a single layer be the
same size as one of the larger towels folded in two)

hot and cold water

Please note again, *this method cannot be self-applied,
help is needed.*

Method

1 The person to be treated undresses and lies down,
face upwards, between the sheets and under one
of the blankets.

2 Immerse the two bath towels in hot water and
wring out. Turn back the blanket and top sheet and
place the hot towels, folded (to make 4 layers) onto
the trunk, so that they cover from side to side and
from shoulders to hips.

3 Cover with the sheet and blanket and leave for
5 minutes.

4 Rinse one of the single-layer (small towels in cold
water, the other in hot. Wring out.

5 Turn back the top sheet and blanket. Place the 'new' (small) hot towel on top of the 'old' (large) hot towels and 'flip' so that small hot towel is directly on the skin. Remove the old towels. Immediately place the small cold towel onto the small hot towel and flip again, so that the cold is next to the skin. Remove small hot towel.

6 Cover with the sheet and blanket and leave for 10 minutes or until the cold towel is warmed.

7 Remove previously cold (now warmed by body heat) towel. The person being treated should now turn over onto his stomach.

8 Repeat steps 2 to 6 for the back.

Notes

If using a bed, take precautions (such as plastic sheeting) not to get this wet.

'Hot' water in this context is of a temperature high enough to prevent you leaving your hand in it for more than 5 seconds.

The coldest water from a running tap is adequate for the 'cold' towel. If it is a hot summer's day, adding ice to the water is acceptable, so long as the resulting temperature contrast is acceptable to the patient.

If the person being treated feels cold after the cold towel is placed, use back, foot or hand massage – through the blanket and towel and/or use visualization – ask the person being treated to think of a sunny beach, for example.

Most importantly, varying the differential between hot and cold – making it a small difference for someone whose immune function and overall degree of vulnerability is poor, for example, and using a large contrast, very hot and very cold, for someone whose constitution is robust – allows for this method to be used on anyone at all.

Exercises

Another important aid to improving the health of this part of the body is exercise. Bending and stretching are especially beneficial as this helps to reduce any muscular stiffness and congestion. Brisk walking every day is also a good idea for circulatory enhancement.

Yoga-type exercises in particular are helpful, and those which safely invert the body (the shoulder stand, for example, or the plough position) are highly recommended. Initially at least these should only be undertaken with the supervision of a qualified yoga instructor.

Some simple yoga postures which can be practised and are helpful in improving prostate drainage and circulation are outlined below.

The first is a very simple kneeling pose. This is easy to achieve unless there are problems with the knees and hips, in which case it should not be attempted. Before doing the postures, remove your shoes and any clothes that might be constricting. Make sure that the floor is not too hard – use a rug or a carpeted floor – and that the room is warm.

Exercise Position 1

Sit on your heels, keeping your back straight. Breathe deeply and relax, then slowly allow your feet to separate so that your buttocks sink between them until they rest on the floor. Breathe deeply several times, allowing the muscles of the legs to relax completely as you breathe out. Keep the spine straight all the time. This has a stimulating effect on the circulation to the pelvic region and should be maintained for a minute or two. Repeat the position daily.

Exercise Position 2

The next pose is one which requires a little practice. Lie on your back on the floor (don't put a cushion under your head), then let your arms extend sideways at an angle of about 45 degrees to the rest of your body, with your palms flat on the floor. Place the soles of your feet together and draw your legs upwards, bending at the knees and allowing their weight to make them spread apart as the soles of your feet are brought higher. As you lift your legs, your buttocks will ease off the floor. This is the upper limit of the pose and should be held for a minute or so. Breathe deeply and slowly all the while, until you feel you wish to roll back downwards to lie flat on the floor. If it is difficult to maintain the position once the buttocks have left the floor, place a small cushion under the buttocks to help to support the position.

In this position of inverted gravity (i.e. the pelvic organs are hanging upside down, so to speak) and with the legs spread as they should be, there is a release of pressure on the pelvic floor which benefits the prostate. This posture should be performed daily.

Exercise Position 3

This is an alternative to Position 2. Kneel on the floor with your weight on your hands and knees. Allow your arms to bend until your forehead rests on the floor and your buttocks are in the air. In this position – which once again inverts the internal organs and releases pressure from the pelvic floor – breathe deeply and at the same time retract your abdomen, i.e. pull your tummy in and up, as though the umbilicus (navel) is being drawn towards the spine. Hold this position and your breath for a few seconds, then release your breath and allow your abdomen to relax again. Repeat 10 times. When you have completed the exercise, sit for a while on your haunches before rising, as you may feel dizzy. (This is true for all the floor exercises, especially if accompanied by deep breathing.)

Please note: Anyone with glaucoma or high blood pressure should avoid this posture until advice is sought from an expert as to its desirability.

These methods are suggested as part of a general attempt to improve abdominal muscle tone and pelvic circulation. There are many other yoga poses, and these may be studied from books or by attending classes.

Traditional Chinese Medicine (Qigong) Prostate Exercises

1 *Buttock-vibrating exercise:* lying on your back with your legs straight, alternately tighten and relax the buttocks as fast as possible so that your hips jiggle up and down; continue until the muscles are tired. There is a direct link between the blood vessels in some of the muscles of the buttocks and the blood vessels which feed and drain the prostate (and the uterus in women). By rapidly contracting these muscles as described, a 'pumping' action is achieved which helps drainage – most important in BPH, when this area is congested.

2 *Pelvic tightening:* lying on your back with your legs bent up so that your feet are near your buttocks, and using your shoulders and feet for support, lift your hips high off the bed or floor, consciously constrict the anus and inhale, then exhale and release the anal contraction, allowing your hips to drop back down

to the bed or floor. Repeat 10 to 20 times. This also 'pumps' the circulation of the area.

3 *Goldfish exercise:* lying on your back with your legs extended, lift your buttocks a fraction off the floor and sway your waist to one side then the other like a fish swimming. Repeat 50 times.

4 *Bicycling exercise:* lying on your back, feet in the air and hands supporting your hips, pedal as though riding a bike, for 2 to 3 minutes.

Prostate Self-help with Reflex Pressure Points

Osteopathic research has shown that certain areas of the body's surface can be felt to change in texture, and to become sensitive to pressure, in response to various problems of the internal organs. When the prostate is disturbed there are two main reflex areas which become sensitive in this way. The first is an area on the outer thigh, about a third of the way between the hip and the knee, which will usually be found to be tight. It has been described as feeling like an 'ensheathing callus'. When this is found (it may extend for some 15 cm or more in this region) and is sensitive to moderate pressure, it probably indicates lymphatic congestion of the prostate. (In women the same area is found to be related to uterine dysfunction.) It is possible to confirm the likelihood of this being an active reflex by also palpating the second area, which is at the very base of the spine between the prominent pelvic bone, which lies just to the side of the last vertebrae of the spine, and the spine itself. An area which feels tight and sensitive in this region, accompanied by sensitivity in the area on the outer thigh, is a confirmation of some reflex activity from the prostate (or uterus). These areas or points are known as Chapman's reflexes, after the osteopathic physician who charted them in the 1930s, or as neurolymphatic reflexes (*see Figure 4*).

Treatment of these points or areas involves the application of moderate pressure first to the leg area, and then to the back area. A period of about 20 seconds of thumb pressure should be given at the tenderest part of the reflex area on the legs. Both legs should be treated in this way if both are found to contain tender reflex points in this region. This should be followed by a similar period of pressure on the reflex areas on the back (both sides of the spine if both are tender to pressure).

It has been shown that the effect of this application of pressure is to reduce the lymphatic congestion in whichever area the points relate to, in this instance the prostate gland. Lymphatic congestion indicates that circulation and drainage of the area is inadequate, and that there may be inflammation. Obviously this reflex stimulus will not cure the condition, but it will certainly help to reduce local swelling and may

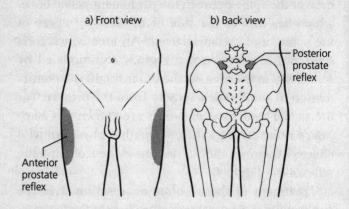

a) Front view   b) Back view

Posterior prostate reflex

Anterior prostate reflex

Figure 4 Neurolymphatic (Chapman's) reflexes

instigate symptomatic relief of the condition, at least for a while. This should therefore be seen as a means by which a degree of first aid may be given while long-term measures (such as diet) are being used.

In order to avoid irritating the local tissues this method should not be applied more than once daily, and only when the reflex area is found to be sensitive. Doing more will not achieve better results, as it is possible both to exhaust a reflex and to irritate it. If it is found to be difficult to press on the points at the side of the base of the spine, then lying face-up on the floor and placing a golf (or tennis) ball strategically under the point will allow for the appropriate degree of pressure to be applied.

This method can also be seen to be diagnostic and prognostic (telling you how the condition is progressing), since if lymphatic drainage improves (using the hydrotherapy methods, dietary changes, etc.) then these reflexes will no longer be tender. (For a deeper understanding of neurolymphatic reflexes as they affect other parts of the body, my book *Modern Neuromuscular Techniques* [Churchill Livingstone] should be consulted.)

Structure and function are inextricably linked, and we must use both, via these methods, to enhance the health of the region as a whole, and the prostate in particular. It is to be hoped that the methods discussed, especially the hydrotherapy measures, are not skipped over as being quaint relics of the past. There is ample evidence of their effectiveness, sometimes dramatically so. This effectiveness should never, however, be seen as sufficient to allow the nutritional measures which are presented in the following chapters to be ignored. The nutritional aspect of prostate problems is the key to recovery.

6
Zinc and the Prostate

Zinc is arguably the single most important element in any approach aimed at improving the condition of the prostate. A major study undertaken in the US on the relationship between zinc and the health of the prostate gland involved assessing the presence of zinc in various tissues of the body. Some 750 patients took part in the trials. Samples of blood were obtained and these were analysed, and the zinc levels determined. Samples of semen were examined and again zinc levels determined. Finally, prostatic tissue itself was obtained, and zinc levels in these structures established.

The results confirmed that determination of zinc levels by the methods used was reliable, and that the results could be reproduced. The level of zinc found in the sperm was found to be a good indicator of the level of zinc concentration found in the prostate gland; this is important since it is not desirable to have to remove small parts of the gland in order to assess the zinc status of the patient. Sperm evaluation proved to be just as accurate as evaluation of the actual tissues of the gland.

The overall results of the study of tissues showed that nearly 40 per cent of the males involved had borderline, or actual, zinc deficiency in the prostate. Those patients who had chronic prostatitis were almost inevitably low in zinc, in both the prostate and sperm analysis, and yet showed normal blood levels of the mineral. A supplement of zinc taken for between 2 and 16 weeks produced symptomatic relief in 70 per cent of the patients. The levels of zinc in the tissues discussed were shown to rise steadily while patients were on supplements.

In patients with cancer of the prostate there was again evidence of zinc deficiency in both sperm and the gland. When there was widespread dissemination of the cancer, the level of zinc in the blood was also shown to be low, but otherwise blood samples showed normal levels of zinc. This indicates that under usual conditions the assessment of zinc by taking a sample of blood is meaningless, insofar as the amounts present in the prostate structures and tissues is concerned.

In cases of prostate enlargement (BPH), where the size of the gland can increase from walnut size to the size of a medium orange, the blood levels were again shown to be normal as far as zinc was concerned, even when local tissues showed a deficit. When supplementation of zinc was carried out in BPH patients the serum levels stayed much the same, but the concentrations in the prostate and sperm increased markedly. These patients also displayed long-term improvement in their condition, as assessed by symptoms being reduced. There was observable shrinkage of the prostate, as assessed by palpation, X-ray examination, and direct observation using an endoscope, in the majority of these patients.

The report on these studies concluded thus:

Zinc may play a specific role in the pathophysiology and treatment of genitourinary diseases. Although zinc has been used as a therapeutic agent in wound healing, chronic ulcers, burns and hepatitis, it has not previously been utilized in a systematic manner, specifically for prostatic diseases.

And yet others had noted many of these findings previously; indeed the connection between prostate and zinc has been known for half a century or more. As Dr Carl Pfeiffer points out in his classic book, *Mental and Elemental Nutrients*. 'Zinc is important for the formation of active sperm in all mammalian species, including man. The prostate and the prostatic secretions are high in zinc.' Dr Pfeiffer also points out that where inflammation of the prostate (prostatis) exists, the local zinc levels often drop to as low as one-tenth of normal levels.

Dr Irving Bush, of the Center for Studies of Prostate Diseases, found that zinc supplementation abolished symptoms in the majority of men suffering from non-infective chronic prostatitis. Dr Kurt Donsbach of California has stated: 'A diseased prostate gland has a very low concentration of zinc, and for some reason vitamin C seems to be more potent, as an anti-infective agent, in the presence of zinc.' (We shall be considering the role of vitamin C later.)

The question obviously is how can we increase zinc levels through diet? Or in other words, which foods contain significant amounts of zinc? This is important since it is patently undesirable to have to take large doses of any substance for unlimited, or very long periods, although in the short term this is probably the only way of boosting levels speedily.

The main food sources are as follows:

Milligrams of zinc per 100 grams (3 ounces) of food:

Peas	4.0
Carrots	2.0
Beets	0.93
Cabbage	0.80
Oysters	143.0

Herrings	100.0
Clams	20.0
Wheat bran	14.0
Whole oatmeal	14.0
Brown rice	2.5
Dates	0.34
Bananas	0.28
Nuts	3.0
Whole wheat	1.04
Refined wheat	0.12
Egg	1.2
Cow's milk	Between 17 and 66
Human milk	Between 2 and 138
Human colostrum (present in first feed to the baby)	Between 70 and 900+
Pumpkin seeds, Sunflower seeds	Over 25

It is interesting to note the large variables in mothers' milk. Researchers such as Dr Pfeiffer suggest zinc supplementation for expectant mothers, since the first feed from the mother containing the colostrum should have a high level of zinc to counteract the high levels of copper with which a baby is born. It has even been suggested that the first seeds of later prostate trouble are sown shortly after birth, if the mother is low in zinc, or if no breast-feeding occurs.

The daily requirement of zinc, in normal health, is around 15 milligrams (mg). However it is important to remember that daily requirements vary from person to person. Some nutrients are required in greater quantities by one individual as compared to another, and these differences need not be small but may vary by a factor of 7 or more. Thus one person may require 10 to 15 mg of zinc daily, in order to remain healthy, and another may require 50 to 100 mg of the same nutrient. These differences are inborn and cannot be changed, nor can they, unfortunately, be easily recognized until problems arise in those who have great needs which are not being met.

We also require more zinc in different circumstances, for example during periods of rapid growth, during puberty, during pregnancy, during all periods of stress and infection, in response to frequent sex (or masturbation). In all such cases the body requires more zinc than normal.

In order to utilize the zinc which is present, the body requires all other nutrients in a balanced form. Specifically, zinc interacts with certain nutrients such as vitamin A, calcium, phosphorus and vitamin C, and is better utilized when these are present in adequate quantities. In particular, zinc has a relationship with a B vitamin called pyridoxine (formerly known as vitamin B_6). If zinc is taken as a supplement, as suggested later, it is important that there are sufficient levels of vitamin B_6 and other nutrients for the zinc to be able to produce beneficial effects.

What can zinc do for the prostate and for sexual function? Pfeiffer puts it thus:

> Zinc will do many things to lubricate the sexual machinery, such as,
> 1. increase penis and testes size in young growing males;
> 2. increase sperm motility;
> 3. decrease prostatitis and normalize secretions;
> 4. replace the zinc loss occasioned by excessive prostate secretion as in sexual foreplay, and replace the zinc lost in the ejaculate;
> 5. help prevent impotency.

However, he cautions that: 'With all this knowledge we still cannot say that anyone's sex life would be better with excess zinc; we can only say that zinc is needed for normal sex activity, normal reproduction, and the perfection of babies of all species.'

Not only men need zinc, of course, for as indicated it is a vital element in breast milk, and is used by the body in large amounts during pregnancy. Pfeiffer points out that it is a vital factor in the health and production of the ova (the female egg). Vaginal secretions are also high in zinc.

Thus the tradition of eating oysters for fertility and

sexual health is seen to be well founded in respect of their zinc content. Consumption of pumpkin seeds is a cheaper way of achieving a similar effect. Dr Donsbach states: 'Folk medicine in many countries of Europe tells us that the men of Bulgaria, Ukraine and Turkey were well aware of the fact that eating a handful of pumpkin seeds daily would prevent prostate problems, and thus enhance their virility.' It is suggested that such seeds contain not only abundant zinc, but other substances, including plant hormones, which benefit man. They also contain desirable forms of essential fatty acids, which we will consider in Chapter 7.

The best forms of zinc to take as a supplement are thought to be zinc orotate or zinc picolinate. This combines the zinc with a substance called orotic acid, which aids its absorption and transportation. Tablets of zinc orotate are in strengths of 100 mg. This is not all zinc, though, for that would represent an excessive intake. Rather it is about 15 per cent zinc and the rest is orotic acid. This provides the daily intake requirement with each tablet, and together with a good supply of zinc from selected foods, as mentioned above, this should replenish stocks of zinc rapidly. As an alternative to zinc orotate, 50 mg daily of zinc picolinate may be taken.

One note of caution: excessive zinc intake competes in the gut for absorption with iron and copper, and long-term zinc supplementation might decrease levels of these important substances. Thus supplementation should be carried out every other day or on 5 or 6 days weekly, ideally at the same time as ensuring an abundant supply of zinc from food such as sunflower and pumpkin seeds, herrings, etc. The nutrients vitamin B_6 and vitamin C should be taken as well; the correct doses of these will be given later in the book. Although the importance of zinc is indisputable, it is essential that other nutrients are not neglected.

7

Fats and Essential Fatty Acids: Their Effects on the Prostate

Modern man consumes a phenomenal amount of fat. Unfortunately this fat is largely made up of a type of fat, called saturated fat, which is considered to be highly detrimental to health. The type of meat eaten and the amount of dairy produce consumed seem to be largely responsible for this, and the role these elements have played in man's diet has changed dramatically in the past century (as, incidentally, has the incidence of prostate hypertrophy and prostate cancer). Another factor which has altered is the way in which animals are reared for consumption. The trend until recently has been for a far higher fat content, although growing awareness seems now to be leading away from this trend.

Leading health authorities, world wide, have told us that no more than 30 per cent of our total energy intake should be derived from fats, and that no more than half of this should be in the form of saturated fats. At present the intake of fats in the Western world is around 40 per cent of total energy consumption, and the ratio between saturated and polyunsaturated fats (the more desirable type) shows that in the UK we eat nearly four times as much saturated as unsaturated fat (instead of equal amounts).

The consequences for health and disease of all this is very important indeed, relating as it does to coronary heart disease, diabetes, gall bladder disease and cancer. It also relates to prostate problems.

In primitive times fat consumption was around 20 per cent of total energy intake, and even the type of fat consumed was different, since free-living animals (game) contain only about 4 per cent of their total body weight as fat (most of this being unsaturated fat) as compared to some 30 per cent of body weight comprising fat in modern beef cattle (and most of this being saturated fat). These are the changes which have contributed to the epidemic proportions of some of the diseases mentioned, as well as to prostate disease.

As mentioned previously, we share prostate problems with our close friend the dog. Experiments in the US at Rutgers University showed that elderly dogs with prostate problems could be helped considerably, with reduction in the size of the prostate, by reducing the cholesterol levels in their blood. Cholesterol levels in the body relate to both a high saturated fat and a high sugar content of the diet.

Examination of human prostates after death in 100 men with BPH, showed that these glands contained 80 per cent more cholesterol on average than normal prostate glands.

Observation in rural Africa shows that people on a low-fat diet had low prostate risk. When the same people changed to a Western dietary pattern, with a high fat (and sugar) content, the production of hormones associated with high incidence of prostate problems rose dramatically.

When similar trials were carried out in reverse in the US, while males with a normally high fat intake and associated production of undesirably high levels of these hormones were shown to reverse this trend when placed, for just a matter of weeks, on a low-fat diet. This was seen as evidence of a reduced risk of prostate cancer in the men whose diet was low in fat.

In order to reduce the incidence of prostate enlargement and specifically of prostate cancer, there should be a major effort directed at reducing both fat intake, altering fat type, and reducing sugar intake. All of these factors are interrelated in the development of high cholesterol levels in the blood, and ultimately in the prostate. This calls for a reduction in the eating of meat derived from domesticated farmed animals such as cattle, pig, sheep, etc. It also means avoiding fried food and the skin on chicken. Dairy produce such as milk, full-fat cheese and butter also come under suspicion and should be reduced drastically.

This leaves fish, poultry (apart from the skin), low-fat dairy produce such as skimmed milk, low-fat cheese such as feta and edam, and low-fat yoghurt (margarines which are not high in polyunsaturated fats, and butter, however, should be avoided), meat as long as it is game (such as rabbit, hare, deer), vegetables, fruit, grains, pulses – all of which would be included in a healthy diet.

However, it has been shown, as previously commented, that sugar also increases cholesterol levels in the blood, and so consumption of this should be reduced to minimal levels too. No white or brown sugar products should be eaten, including cakes, sweets, pastries as well as sugar itself, if prostate problems are to be avoided. We obtain ample natural sugar from our fruit and vegetable intake, and the refined sugars present in so many foods are harmful in a number of respects, not least being the promotion of heart problems, cancer and obesity.

A diet rich in fibre is a must. Fibre is best obtained simply by eating abundant vegetables and fruits, as well as foods derived from the pulse family (lentils, chickpeas, beans, etc).

The combination of a diet low in saturated fats, high in fibre, and low in sugar is the key to health in general and prostate health in particular.

In addition we must ensure an adequate intake of those fats which are useful, the essential fatty acids. These have a beneficial effect on the prostate and on health in general.

Essential Fatty Acids and the Prostate

In the early 1940s two doctors in California noticed that some of the patients to whom they were giving high dosages of vitamin F (another name for essential fatty acids or EFAs) were showing marked improvements in the status of their enlarged prostates. Drs Hart and Cooper went on to conduct a clinical trial on some 20 patients using this approach. This is what they did: They palpated the size of the enlarged prostate of each participant in the trial; took a sample of urine as well as a detailed record of symptoms such as urinary problems, including weakness of the urine stream, dribbling, passing water during the night and cystitis (bladder inflammation). The patients were all given thorough investigations to exclude the possibility of other factors such as hormone or nutrient imbalances. Blood samples were taken to note the various levels of fats and other substances. Hormone levels were monitored and the patients were then placed on vitamin F (essential fatty acid) supplementation.

Re-examination was carried out at monthly intervals at which time all procedures, as described above, were repeated. The patients also reported weekly on any changes which they had noted.

The results were very impressive indeed. All cases showed a reduction in the amount of urine left in the bladder after the individual had passed water. This residual urine makes the bladder prone to infection, as the stagnant urine is an ideal medium for bacteria. In 12 out of the 19 patients who completed the trial there was a complete absence of residual urine at the end of the treatment period, and consequently an absence of previously noted cystitis. In 13 of the cases there was elimination of the need to pass water during the night. There was, in all patients, a decrease in fatigue and leg pains, as well as an increase in sexual interest. Dribbling was eliminated in 18 of the 19 patients, and the force of the urine stream increased. In all cases there was a rapid reduction in the size of the prostate, confirmed by palpation.

All the patients showed enthusiasm over the improvement in their physical well-being. Those who showed less improvement than the others all had a history of gonorrhoeal infection in the past.

The beneficial effects of the essential fatty acids do not stop with the prostate. They aid in preventing cholesterol deposits forming in the arteries; they promote healthy skin and hair; they protect against the harmful effects of X-rays; they improve and support glandular function and help to ensure calcium availability to cells; they combat cardiovascular disease and assist in the burning (metabolizing) of saturated fats, thus reducing their harmful potential and assisting in weight reduction.

There are numerous safe sources of essential fatty acids. Among the best of these are linseed oil (flax seed), sunflower and pumpkin seeds. EFAs are also plentiful in walnuts, almonds, pecan nuts and avocado pears (note that brazil and cashew nuts do not have a high level of EFA). Eating a fresh salad every day garnished with sunflower seeds and fresh nuts, or sprinkling linseed on to a bowl of cereal will supply an adequate amount of EFA to your diet. The body can manufacture the other essential fatty acids if sufficient linoleic acid, which is found in a wide range of foods, including vegetables and grains, is present.

Apart from adding foods high in these oils to the diet, it is possible to obtain them by taking supplements specifically formulated to supply the right quantities and types of fatty acids. It is advisable to take such supplements with vitamin E, in supplement form, and to do so at mealtimes. It is also important to be aware that the more carbohydrate consumed, the more essential fatty acids the body requires. A daily supplement of linseed oil (be sure to obtain a form which is designed for human consumption) at a rate of 1 to 2 tablespoons of the oil daily is recommended. Evening Primrose oil is available in health food stores.

This is an excellent if slightly expensive way of obtaining EFAs; 500 to 1,000 mg daily (one or two capsules) of this should be taken. On the other hand, an inexpensive way of obtaining adequate supplies is to eat a handful of pumpkin and/or sunflower seeds, twice daily.

By avoiding excessive saturated fat (meat, dairy products, etc.) and sugars, and by ensuring adequate intake of EFAs as laid out here, a major contribution will be made to general health and to prostate well-being.

We will now consider other nutrients and substances, such as pollen and ginseng, as well as the role of protein and particular amino acids in the prevention and safe treatment of prostate problems.

8
Nutrient Therapies for Prostate Problems

Amino Acids (Protein Fractions) and the Prostate

We have already seen that there is strong evidence that a high-protein diet acts to protect against prostate enlargement. As with most of the body's structures, the cells which compose the prostate gland are largely constructed of protein. Cells of glandular structures such as the prostate, however, have a uniquely high-protein component. This is one reason why these are often the parts of animals which are eaten first, from choice, by predators and by primitive hunter-gatherer peoples. Such peoples choose to eat the organs such as the spleen, liver and glands before bothering to eat the muscle meats which are so much the dominant choice of Western man. Predators make similar choices, leaving the muscle meat to last, or to animals such as hyenas and vultures.

The ratios of the various building blocks of protein which make up the particular cells of different glands varies, as would be expected, thus imparting the unique characteristics of each gland or organ. It is conceivable that a very high-protein diet provides the particular amino acids needed to protect the health of the prostate. This type of diet is close to that followed by hunter-gatherer peoples, who also consume large amounts of plant food and thus avoid the over-acidification of the body which could result from excessive protein intake.

An alternative to the consumption of huge amounts of protein is, however, readily available. This involves supplementing the diet with three specific amino acids (out of the 20 there are in total), in order to achieve remarkable benefits to enlarged prostate conditions.

A report appeared as long ago as 1958, in the *Journal of the Maine Medical Association*, which described an important trial using these three amino acids – glycine, alanine, and glutamic acid – in combination. The trial involved 45 men who all had BPH (benign prostatic hypertrophy) with a range of symptoms which included discomfort, night-time urgency, delayed urination (an inability to begin to pass water when this was desired), frequency of urination and uncontrollable urgency. These patients varied in age from 37 to 75, and most had had the complaint for at least four years. One group of the men were given a supplement of these three amino acids; the other received a placebo (a dummy tablet). The tablets (supplements or placebo) were taken after meals for three months.

The results were startling. Of those who had received the real amino acid tablets, over 90 per cent were found to have a reduction in size of the prostate, and in a third, the prostate had returned to normal size. The need to pass water at night was totally eliminated in three-quarters of these patients, with over 90 per cent reporting a marked improvement in this symptom. Urgency was relieved in 80 per cent of these patients, and almost the same percentage lost the frequency symptoms, with 70 per cent noting absence of the symptom of delayed urination.

Those who had been given the dummy tablets showed no such improvement until they were eventually placed on the amino acid supplementation.

Since there is no danger at all from supplementation using a natural substance such as an amino acid in the dosages used, this was an extremely successful result. Interestingly, a number of other symptoms, including tendency to swellings in various parts of the body, improved at the same time. This symptom is characteristic of protein deficiency, which might well have been the underlying cause, alleviated by the amino acid therapy.

Suggested Dosages

Glycine: 200 mg per day
Glutamic acid: 200 mg per day
Alanine: 200 mg per day

Later research in Japan and the US gave impressive
results as well:

1 In Japan, dysuria (discomfort on passing water)
   was improved in 14 of the 17 patients using the
   amino acids, and residual urine (not being able to
   empty the bladder adequately) was better in 8 of
   the 134 patients with this symptom.
2 In the US, the need to pass water at night was
   improved in 95 per cent of the 45 patients on
   the trial; urgency improved in 80 per cent and
   frequency was reduced by over 70 per cent – and
   none of the patients showed any side-effects at all
   from this treatment.

These three amino acids are available in combination
in the UK, in formulations which match those used in
the trials mentioned, from better health food stores
and some pharmacies.

Pollen and the Prostate

Pollen is rich both in protein and essential fatty acids, and of course in plant hormones, so the benefits found from its use in treating a number of conditions, including prostate enlargement, may be related to the presence of any one of these constituents, or to all of them.

A report in the *Swedish Medical Journal* described the use of pollen extract tablets manufactured by the firm B. Cernelle. Out of 10 patients with BPH, five were relieved of their symptoms and the prostate size returned to normal over a one-year treatment period. The patients with inflamed prostates showed a most marked improvement.

A Japanese trial at Nagasaki University School of Medicine, Department of Urology, used the same pollen extracts on some 30 patients, all suffering from acute prostatitis. The results showed that just over half of the patients, 16 in all, enjoyed results described as 'markedly effective'. Another 13 cases were 'effective', but not as strongly so, and in only one case was there no improvement.

In the Swedish trial, four tablets of pollen (named 'Cernilton') were taken daily; in the Japanese trials a higher intake of six tablets daily was used. In none of the trials was there any report of side-effects.

It seems likely that the combination of fatty acids (*see Chapter 7*), plant hormones and protein present in pollen was responsible for the benefits noted in these two trials.

Another plant used in the treatment of the prostate, and in other conditions, is ginseng.

Ginseng and Prostate Problems

Long employed as an aphrodisiac and general tonic in the Orient, ginseng (*Panax ginseng*) is the powdered root of this remarkable plant. It is known to contain a number of properties, one of which enhances the normal production of the male hormone testosterone. It also decreases prostate weight when administered regularly.

In those suffering from BPH there are abnormal levels of testosterone, with a corresponding drop in the intestinal absorption of zinc. A vicious cycle results which ends ultimately in enlargement of the gland. Ginseng used regularly would appear to provide benefits in terms of all of these negative factors. No clinical trials have been reported, but there is a long tradition of the successful use of ginseng in the Orient and in individual patients in the West. It would seem to provide a useful supportive role whilst more fundamental action is being taken, through the use of added essential fatty acids and zinc, for example.

Twenty drops of the fluid extract of ginseng are taken three times daily as a therapeutic dose. It is important that genuine *Panax ginseng* is obtained, as the demand for this substance has led to a plethora of inferior products reaching the market.

Russian research in particular has resulted in a degree of respectability being granted to the use of ginseng and other remarkable plant substances, like the Siberian eleutherococcus. Such plant substances are known as adaptogens, and are believed to be able to increase the overall capacity of the body to overcome external stresses through adaptation. This has implications relating to the ageing process as well as to factors such as radiation damage (which is in itself an acceleration of the ageing process).

One of the key benefits of adaptogens is that they can enhance the body's ability to utilize oxygen. This in itself is a crucial factor in terms of the ageing process, and therefore is part of the complex of factors negatively affecting prostate function as a man gets older.

All adaptogens work slowly; they do not produce sudden changes, but have to be used for some weeks before any noticeable alteration in symptoms will be felt. Eleutherococcus is at least as powerful an adaptogen as ginseng and these two substances are available generally. However, their popularity has led to cheap imitations being placed on the market, and it is important that only active forms are used. Check sources carefully to ensure that only genuine *Panax ginseng* or Siberian eleutherococcus are used. Health food stores should be able to guide you as to the quality of the adaptogen of your choice.

It is also worth remembering that the use of adaptogens should be seen as just one part of a general approach which includes the nutritional advice already presented. Adaptogens on their own will not produce a complete reversal of a change which involves deficits of crucial nutrients such as zinc and essential fatty acids as described in previous chapters.

Sereno Repens

The fruit of the palm tree (saw palmetto berries, also known as *Serenoa repens* or *Sabal serrulata,* which come from a scrubby palm tree common in and native to Florida) contains oils and fatty acids which act to inhibit various biochemical activities related to the development of BPH. Their action leads to a reduction in the activity of 5-alpha reductase, the overactivity of which helps to increase levels of dihydrotestosterone in the prostate.

Use of Sereno repens has, in trials in humans and animals, been shown to be effective in aiding reduction in the size of the prostate gland in BPH.

Twenty drops of the fluid extract of this plant's berries are taken three times daily as a therapeutic dose. Again this should be accompanied by the use of nutritional support in the way of protein, essential fatty acids and zinc.

Pygeum Africanus

The powdered bark of an African tree has been used for many years to treat prostate problems. French research has shown that it has anti-inflammatory effects as well as lowering cholesterol levels – both of which may explain why it is helpful in treatment of the enlarged or inflamed prostate. No side-effects are found. A number of products containing this plant extract are readily available from health food stores or herbal suppliers.

Raw Glandular Extracts and the Prostate

Over the past 50 years or more a science has grown around the use of extracts of glandular substances derived from healthy young animals. These glands secrete hormonal substances in the animal, and they are remarkably similar to the glands found in humans. It has been found that depending upon the method of extraction and preservation of such glandular substances, they can have a profound effect on the human body by supplying it with the essential raw materials contained within the glands. The body is able to utilize these to its benefit in many conditions, including prostate enlargement.

The glands, which interact within what is known as the endocrine system, include the pituitary, thymus, pineal, hypothalamus, thyroid and parathyroid, adrenals, kidney, pancreas and the gonads or sex glands. Imbalances between hormones occur, and other secretions from these various glands become deficient and unbalanced as a consequence of age or ill-health, and especially if there is a lack of a balanced nutritional pattern. It is the rebalancing of these secretions which the use of glandular extracts is designed to achieve.

The most potent method of achieving effects is by injecting such glandular substances. This process often receives publicity when notable personalities are reported as having 'youth-enhancing' therapy via glandular treatment. It is the chance of a degree of youthful regeneration and vitality which has made this such a fashionable and expensive process. However a much less expensive, if moderately less effective, method exists which involves taking glandular extracts orally in tablet or capsule form. It used to be thought that this route was useless, since the digestive process would reduce any hormone or enzyme molecules present into their constituent amino acids, thus making them no more therapeutic than a piece of cheese or an egg. However, recent research has shown that the claims of the endocrinologists who advocated oral use of glandular substances were not far-fetched, since around half of large-molecule substances such as enzymes pass through the digestive process intact. It is also now known that a good proportion of these will reach the tissues of the body intact, as complex proteins. Thus it is noted that such elements of the original tissue, whether hormone, enzyme, polypeptide, essential fatty acid, etc., can and do reach appropriate tissues and can therefore aid in their regeneration and health enhancement.

The most used of these substances is the extract of thymus gland, which has an effect on the total immune function (defence system) of the body, and which influences all other glandular centres in the body. Other tissues are now being used in therapeutic settings, and where appropriate some, such as liver, stomach, heart, etc., are being provided in tablet form. Sometimes a general mixture of all the available tissues is given in a sort of cocktail which the body can then sort out as its needs dictate. Such a mixture, together with an extract of prostate and/or orchic tissue (testicles), is used in prostate regeneration treatment. It has been found that these are better utilized when a sound general nutritional status exists, and so they should be seen as a part of a general approach, rather than as remedies on their own.

Research has shown that the method of extraction of these glandular substances is critical to their potential value. The methods used include freeze-drying, heat-processing and salt-precipitation. Without going into technical detail, it is apparent to researchers that freeze-drying results in the maximum retention of vital elements. It also avoids removal of the fat content, which is vital for the maintenance of some of the fat-soluble enzymes in these tissues.

Another key element in the value of the extract – especially in this age of BSE – is the source of the animal which has been used to provide the extract. Those derived from areas where BSE is active, as well as those herds exposed to insecticides and hormone treatment, will be either potentially dangerous or sub-standard compared to those not so contaminated. In general it is considered that the extracts derived from New Zealand are safer than others.

Glandulars which are 'buffered' are more likely to pass the initial stages of digestion unscathed, and thus be available for uptake by the body and transportation to the desired site.

Prostate and male glandular formulae are available from specialist health food suppliers. Remember always to check that sources are safe and that methods of manufacture are assessed before the purchase and use of these substances.

The reason for taking orchic tissues relates to the fact that one of the major roles of the testes is to produce testosterone, the hormone which maintains prostate health and size, and which, if deficient, results in enlargement. It is thus desirable that testicular function be enhanced, as well as prostate. If such glandular extracts are taken, it is important that adequate essential fatty acid intake and zinc also be included in the programme, as discussed in Chapter 4.

A normal course of treatment for the use of glandular substances is six weeks, with two tablets of prostate extract being taken after each meal. The course can be repeated after a two-month interval, if still required.

Herbal Help for Prostatitis

Echinacea Angustifolia (Purple Coneflower) and Chimaphilia Umbellata (Pipissewa)

When the problem is not just enlarged prostate (BPH) but an inflamed one as well, there are a number of herbs which can give assistance.

1   *Chimaphilia umbellata* (Pipissewa) is an evergreen plant widely used by herbalists in treating bladder and urinary tract disorders. It has been found to be useful in the treatment of chronic prostatitis. It acts as an antiseptic but should only be used under advice from a health care professional, since self-treatment of prostatitis without supervision is unwise, because of the risks of a wider urinary tract involvement.

2 *Echinacea angustifolia* (Purple Coneflower) is one
 of the most widely used 'natural antibiotics'
 available, and if there exists any active infection
 this herb is probably the most useful. It is widely
 available on its own in liquid and capsule form as
 well as in combination with associated useful herbs
 such as Berberis and Hydrastis.

Note
See also important notes regarding replenishment of
friendly bacteria later in this chapter if antibiotics have
been taken, plus a combined approach (nutrition and
herbs) for dealing with yeast overgrowth, which can be
a major cause of prostatitis.

See also Chapter 9 for a vitamin C approach to
prostatitis.

Summary of Nutrient Supplements for BHP

• Zinc – as an orotate or picolinate: if zinc orotate is
 taken, the dose is 100 to 200 mg daily for five or six
 days per week, and one tablet of chelated copper on
 alternate days; if zinc picolinate is taken, then
 dosage is 50 mg daily for six days per week for at
 least six months.
• Chelated copper should be taken on alternate days
 (providing 1 mg of copper) to prevent a zinc:copper
 imbalance when supplementing with zinc.

- Pyridoxine (vitamin B_6) – 50 to 100 mg daily.
- Fatty acid supplementation (EFA) – take 1 tablespoon of cold-pressed flaxseed oil twice daily, or two 500-mg capsules of Oil of Evening Primrose.
- Vitamin E in dosages of 200 to 400 iu should be taken daily when EFA supplements are being taken.
- Amino acids – glycine, alanine and glutamic acid, 200 mg of each daily at the same time, away from any other supplements and away from mealtimes.
- Pollen extract – three to six tablets daily.
- Sereno repens – 20 drops of fluid extract to be taken three times daily. This should aim to provide approximately 300 mg (or ml) daily in two doses.
- Panax ginseng – 20 drops of fluid extract to be taken three times daily, or approximately 50 mg if in solid form.
- Raw glandular extracts – prostate and orchic, 2 tablets after each meal for six weeks, every three months.

In all of these measures a period of not less than six months should be considered as a basic time scale.

After this, if results have been satisfactory, a maintenance dosage of zinc and essential fatty acids of about 25 per cent of the therapeutic doses given above is suggested indefinitely.

The nutrients and other substances discussed above are all related to BPH and to prostatitis. One of the major accompanying problems of these conditions is frequent cystitis and urethritis. In order to improve this, a major contribution can be achieved from the judicious use of vitamin C and cranberry extracts as discussed below.

Prostatic Inflammation Problems (Prostatitis), Cystitis and Urethritis

Vitamin C

These notes on vitamin C and prostatitis are a summary of what is presented in more detail in Chapter 9.

It is reported by authorities in the US that effective treatment of urethritis (inflammation of the tube carrying the urine and sperm out of the body) can be achieved by taking 3 or more grams of vitamin C daily for four days.

When there is retention of urine, so common in prostate enlargement, there is a danger of infection and inflammation of the bladder. Chronic cystitis (inflammation of the bladder) can result from decomposition of the ammonia in the urine in such a situation. This increases the tendency for the urine to become more alkaline and less acid, which in turn can result in crystals forming in the urine, causing pain and irritation. The increased acidity in the urine which accompanies high doses of some forms of vitamin C (ascorbic acid) helps to reverse this tendency, relieving the symptoms rapidly and reducing the dangers of infection. Some people take as much as 10 grams of vitamin C daily when cystitis is common, and this achieves the desired results quickly and avoids the dangers of kidney infection (pyelitis) which can result from infection in the urinary tract.

Different types of vitamin C can be acidic or alkaline; details of how to choose appropriately and test for acid levels of the urine are in Chapter 9.

Linus Pauling, twice winner of the Nobel prize and advocate of vitamin C in therapy, maintained that when large amounts of vitamin C are taken as much as 60 per cent of the substance which reaches the bloodstream ends up being voided in the urine. This, though, is not a waste by any means, because of the benefits it brings to the urinary tract (bladder, urethra, etc.). Pauling also claimed that taking vitamin C can dramatically reduce the dangers of bladder cancer.

As mentioned previously, vitamin C acts as an anti-infection agent far more efficiently when it is in the presence of adequate zinc. It thus makes sense that in attempting to normalize prostate problems, including the side-effects of prostate enlargement, urethritis and cystitis, vitamin C should be a major element in the treatment programme.

At least 3 grams of vitamin C should be taken daily in separate doses, during the therapeutic period (six months at least); if there is an active inflammation of the urethra or bladder this can usefully be increased to as much as 10 grams per day until symptoms decrease. This high dosage of vitamin C could result in diarrhoea, which will rapidly be relieved when the vitamin C dose is reduced a little. It is a minor inconvenience, however, compared with the side-effects of drugs commonly used in treating such conditions (*see Chapter 9*).

Cranberry juice reduces the ability of bacteria to adhere to the bladder wall (or that of the urethra) and so when its consumption is accompanied by a high water intake the bacteria are literally flushed out of the system. Most commercial cranberry juice has a high sugar content, however; only sugar-free versions are suggested here.

A better choice, with more rapid effects, is to purchase freeze-dried cranberry juice powder, which all health stores will supply either in capsule or powder form. A teaspoon of this (or several capsules) taken twice daily should rapidly assist in eliminating all but the most stubborn of bladder infections. Using cranberry extracts at the same time as taking high-dosage vitamin C supplementation is safe.

For prostate inflammation consider also the use of *Pygeum africanus*, *Echinacea angustifolia* (Purple

Coneflower) and *Chimaphilia umbellata* (Pipissewa) as discussed earlier in this chapter.

Note
See also important notes regarding replenishment of friendly bacteria later in this chapter.

Nutritional Sources of Vitamins, Minerals and EFA

In Chapter 10 we will consider a dietary pattern which should accompany this type of nutrient therapy. The diet is of course a fundamental source of many of the nutrients discussed and so should be seen as an ongoing concern, not something to use for a while and then abandon. The problems of the prostate are often the result of years of improper diet, among other factors, and the reform of the diet is therefore a basic requirement of prostate health.

The objectives of such a diet should be to deal comprehensively with the provision of the various nutrients already discussed, as well as promoting other factors such as bowel health and cholesterol normality, via a high fibre intake.

Among the foods which should form a major part of the diet (and some which should be avoided) are those summarized below which provide specific nutrients or which influence the biochemistry of the body in ways that assist in helping prostate problems.

Therapeutic Foods

- Omega-3 and omega-6 fatty acids: vegetables, nuts, seed oils, salmon, herring, mackerel, sardines, walnuts, flaxseed oil, evening primrose oil, blackcurrant oil
- Foods which assist in balancing hormone levels: apples, cherries, olives, plums, carrots, yams, tomatoes, potatoes, peppers, aubergines (eggplant), peanuts, soy products, coconut, brown rice, barley, oats, wheat
- Foods rich in zinc and vitamin E: squash seeds, almonds, sesame seeds, tahini, kelp, raw pumpkin seeds, sunflower seeds (note – eating at least 25 such seeds several times a day would be required to influence zinc levels significantly), tangerines, cherries, figs, lychee, mangoes, seaweeds
- High-fibre foods – which means all vegetables, whole grains, unpolished rice, fruits

Avoid
- alcohol – especially beer
- saturated fats
- strong spices, spicy food

- dairy products
- fatty foods, fried foods
- coffee, caffeine.

(See also the notes on diet under the heading 'Three month basic anti-Candida strategy', page 101.)

Probiotic Supplementation – General Background Information

For assistance on controlling yeast overgrowth (Candida, *see Chapter 2*) or for intestinal problems (constipation, for example) or for replenishment of important bowel flora after antibiotic therapy, probiotic supplementation is extremely helpful and important.

The three bacteria mentioned in these notes are:

1 *Lactobacillus acidophilus*, which lives in the small intestine and which helps to detoxify the local environment, recycle and balance cholesterol and hormones, and manufacture specific B vitamins.
2 *Bifidobacteria*, which live in the large bowel – the colon – and perform roles similar to those of *L. acidophilus*.
3 *L. bulgaricus* – not normally found in the human gut but a bacteria with enormously helpful habits, among them killing yeasts and unfriendly bacteria.

L. bulgaricus is also one of the bacteria which can turn milk into yoghurt (the other is *thermophilus*). Bulgaricus is known as a 'bifidogenic' bacteria, which means that it helps the other friendly bacteria to colonize the digestive tract, where it remains after being swallowed for about three weeks. We cannot live without the first two bacteria discussed, especially as they offer our main controls over disease-causing yeasts and bacteria in the gut.

The conditions which damage the friendly bacteria most are bowel toxicity (stasis, constipation) anti-biotics, and a high-sugar/high-fat diet.

Probiotic supplements maintain their potency for much longer periods when not exposed to heat or moisture. Keep all probiotic supplements refrigerated for long-term storage. For therapeutic dosages, avoid liquids and gelatin capsules, which have a high moisture content, as this causes the probiotics to lose their potency rapidly – pure powdered freeze-dried bacterial cultures are best.

Mix probiotic products in unchlorinated, tepid water to maintain optimum viability of the cells before consuming.

Gradually build-up to therapeutic dosage levels to prevent rapid, sometimes uncomfortable, changes in intestinal ecology which can lead to gas.

For best results, *L. acidophilus* and *Bifidobacterium bifidum* should be taken on an empty stomach, 30 to 45 minutes before meals. *L. bulgaricus* should be taken with or immediately following meals.

Caution

People with milk intolerance may not be able to use milk-based products. If the condition is a simple lactose intolerance, most patients will do very well on a milk-based *L. acidophilus* supplement. The production of lactase as a by-product of *L. acidophilus* metabolism has been shown to be effective in the management of lactose intolerance. With more sensitive patients, the use of a milk-free *L. acidophilus* supplements for a month or two may improve a lactose intolerance enough to allow for a milk-based supplement to be tolerated.

Adult Dosages

- During and following antibiotic therapy – ½ to 1 teaspoon *L. acidophilus* three times a day before meals. It is recommended that *Bifidobacterium bifidum* also be taken, ½ to 1 teaspoon three times a day before meals, for optimum results.

  If possible, take probiotic supplements at a different time of the day than antibiotics, if you are currently taking these. Continue supplementation for a month at therapeutic levels after discontinuation of antibiotics.

- Acute intestinal distress: 1 teaspoon of both *L. acidophilus* and *Bifidobacterium bifidum* every hour until symptoms cease.
- Chronic constipation (important to normalize where BPH exists): 2½ teaspoons *L. bulgaricus* two to three times per day with meals for several weeks. Follow with maintenance dosages of *L. acidophilus* and *Bifidobacterium bifidum*.
- Candidiasis: Oral administration – 1 teaspoon of both *L. acidophilus* and *Bifidobacterium bifidum* three times a day before meals.

  It is recommended that 2–3 teaspoons of *L. bulgaricus* three times per day with meals be added to this protocol for several weeks.

  If severe Candida 'die-off' symptoms occur, reduce dosage and then gradually increase again.

- Local application if there is chronic bowel problems or chronic Candida overgrowth (*see Candida questionnaire, Chapter 2*): Fill two large-size or four small-size gelatin capsules with *L. acidophilus* and insert rectally before bedtime, for 10 days. Or, mix 1 rounded teaspoon of *L. acidophilus* with 2 tablespoons of plain regular yoghurt (not low- or non-fat). Insert rectally before bedtime, for 10 days.

Note: Do not fill capsules ahead of time, as the high moisture content may destroy the viability of the *acidophilus*. Empty two-piece gelatin capsules are available at most health food stores and pharmacies.

Maintenance dosages when symptoms are under control: ¾ teaspoon *L. acidophilus* and ¼ teaspoon *Bifidobacterium bifidum* once daily, on an empty stomach.

Note: Lacto-vegetarians, athletes and those of African or East Asian ancestry may have a need for more *Bifidobacterium bifidum* than *L. acidophilus* due to their high intake of complex carbohydrates or inherited factors: ¾ teaspoon *Bifidobacterium bifidum* and ¼ teaspoon *L. acidophilus*, once daily.

Three-month Basic Anti-Candida Strategy

Ideally to be undertaken only under supervision of an appropriately qualified and licensed health care professional (to accompany other strategies for treating prostate problems, as appropriate).

1 Caprylic acid (coconut plant extract) – 1 capsule with each meal (that is, three times a day). Acts as an antifungal.
2 Biotin – 500 microgrammes (mcg) twice daily. This B vitamin helps to control the yeast's tendency to alter to a more aggressive form.

3 High-potency garlic – 1 capsule with each meal
   (three times a day). Antifungal, antibiotic.
4 Either any of the following three herbs, individually
   or in combination:
   Hydrastis canandensis (Goldenseal)
   Berberis vulgaris (Barberry) and/or
   Echinacea angustifolia (Purple Coneflower)
   – three times daily as an antifungal, antibacterial,
   immune-enhancing support
   and/or
   Pau D'arco tea – three to four times daily.

These herbs should be obtained from a reputable
herbal supplier or health food store and used
according to the instructions on the pack.

Encouraging Repopulation of Intestinal Flora

5 High-quality *acidophilus* and *Bifidobacteria*
   (powder or capsule form) – between meals (three
   times daily), either a capsule of each, or between
   one-quarter and a whole teaspoon of powdered
   versions of each (*see notes earlier in this chapter*).
   Also *L. bulgaricus* as discussed above.
6 General nutritional support is useful – taking a
   well-formulated, yeast-free, hypoallergenic,
   multivitamin/multimineral to provide at least the
   recommended daily allowance of major nutrients.

Dietary Suggestions for Candida

- Chew well/eat slowly/try not to drink much with meals.
- Eat three small main meals daily as well as two snack meals where possible (no sugar-rich food) or take 3 to 5 grams of full-spectrum amino acid complex between main meals, twice daily.
- Include in the diet as much ginger, cinnamon and garlic (as well as other aromatic herbs such as oregano) as possible – all are antifungal and most also aid digestive processes.
- To assist with bowel function, regularly (daily, same time of day) take at least 1 tablespoonful of linseed. Swallow with water, unchewed to provide a soft fibre to assist intestinal emptying.
- **Avoid as far as possible all refined sugars** and for the first few weeks avoid very sweet fruit as well (melon, sweet grapes). Avoid aged cheeses, dried fruits and any food obviously derived from or containing yeast (in case of sensitization).
- Avoid caffeine (coffee, tea, chocolate, cola. etc.) as this produces a sugar release which is not desirable where yeast has proliferated.
- Avoid alcohol
- If possible avoid all yeast-based foods – including bread and anything that has contained yeast in its manufacture or which might contain mould.

You may feel off-colour for the first week of such a programme as yeast 'die-off' takes place.

Note
Many other antifungal substances are available and may be more effective in certain cases than the suggestions above, which are however usually beneficial if the programme is maintained for several months.

9
Inflammation of the Prostate: The Vitamin C Strategy

Our major consideration so far has been enlargement of the prostate (BPH) and its consequences. In passing we have looked at some of the methods in which an inflamed or infected prostate (prostatitis) might be helped, but now we will concentrate on a particularly effective but somewhat complicated aspect of inflammation or infection, since this represents a more aggravating development than simple prostate enlargement.

As has already been shown there are a number of ways in which inflammation and/or infection can arise. These include the development of crystals of phosphate in the urethra and bladder due to inadequate acidification of the urine. Another cause is the development of bacteria activity in stagnant urine, when the bladder is unable to be emptied efficiently.

This is often combined with decomposition of the ammonia in the bladder urine. There may be primary infection elsewhere, such as in the teeth.

Organisms may multiply in prostatic fluid itself, which normally contains antibacterial elements, but which may not be thus protected at this time because of inadequate nutrient status involving zinc, essential fatty acids and probably vitamin C. Alternatively, intestinal overgrowth of yeast may be involved in the bladder, urethra and prostate. There are also other forms of crystalline development which may occur and produce irritation, if the urine is excessively acidic.

The Prostate and Recurrent Urinary Infections

The questionnaire on page 22 outlines the most common indicators of prostate enlargement (benign prostatic hypertrophy). There is one other sign which should lead to suspicion of prostate enlargement: recurrent urinary tract infections.

If a relapse occurs after appropriate antibiotic therapy, then this may indicate a number of possibilities. Among these are kidney infection, a stone obstructing the free flow of urine, or prostate enlargement which is also obstructing the free flow of urine.

If the prostate is infected with bacteria (chronic bacterial prostatitis), then it becomes a focal point for recurrent infection of the urinary tract (bladder, urethra, etc.). People affected in this way may have no signs of prostate enlargement such as those detailed in the questionnaire, but have recurrent infections, usually involving the same micro-organism. This may recur every few months or more frequently, one infection starting almost as soon as the previous one has cleared up. This requires an accurate diagnosis, and means consulting a health professional who can do cultures as well as examine the prostate as to its status.

One agent which may be involved in prostatitis is trichomonas vaginitis. This is a protozoa and is spread by sexual transmission from an infected person. Its ability to thrive in an individual will depend upon such factors as local tissue acidity and hormone presence. When it is in an optimum environment for growth, and is able to replicate, it produces inflammation of the mucosal lining of the tissues. In women this may involve the vagina; in both sexes it may involve the urethra and/or the bladder; and in males the prostate. Symptoms such as itching, burning and a red-yellow discharge are noted and, depending upon the area, either urethritis or prostatitis (or vaginitis) will be found.

The possibility of infection by trichomonas, or of a yeast such as Candida albicans or a bacteria, should be borne in mind when symptoms such as these are recurrent. If sexually transmitted, then all contacts should be appropriately treated to prevent recurrence. The first and most important task is to identify which micro-organisms are involved in any recurrent infection.

Treatment

Medical treatment of inflammation/infection of the prostate is to attack the bacterial aspect of the problems. This in itself does little apart from stopping the infection for the short term. It is no more a long-term solution than would be killing the flies around a rubbish bin in the vain hope that this would get rid of the rubbish. In other words, it in no way improves the background reasons which allowed the infection to occur. Thus recurrence is more or less assured, and the prospects are less than good for health in the region. Nevertheless because of the risks which infections in this region carry of spreading to the kidneys, the infection needs to be brought under control, as well as the underlying reasons for its existence being dealt with.

If this is not comprehensively done, the long-term prospect is that the individual might well find himself a candidate for surgery to remove the prostate (or develop kidney problems as well as whatever else is being suffered). Prostate surgery is a fairly serious operation and is one which can leave bladder function impaired. In many instances it is an unnecessary operation, because reduction in the size of the prostate is usually not difficult to achieve by means of the methods outlined previously. And once reduction in size is achieved, it will lead eventually to normalization of the bladder-emptying mechanisms, as well as to the correct acidic balance in the urine, thus reducing the chances of infection and of inflammation. This is the logical approach to treating recurrent urethritis and cystitis.

Whether treating an episode of urethritis, cystitis, prostatitis or pyelitis, there is one approach which is always worth attempting because of its excellent results and safety: vitamin C should be taken in very high doses.

Urine Testing

It is possible to obtain from any pharmacist litmus paper or a self-test kit for assessing the acidity of the urine. If the urine shows itself to be excessively acid (a level of 4.8 or lower) rather than the normal levels of acidity which are anywhere between a pH of 5 and a pH of 7 (which is neutral, neither acid nor alkaline), and there has been a diagnosis of stones in the bladder or kidneys, then the vitamin C taken should be in the form of sodium ascorbate, which will not further increase the acidity of the urine.

In such cases it is also suggested that a dose of 100 milligrams (mg) of vitamin B₆ be taken daily.

If the urine tests as alkaline (anywhere from a pH of 7.0 upwards), which is abnormal since it should always be acid, then the vitamin C should be taken in the form of ascorbic acid, rather than sodium ascorbate. This will acidify the urine, and if phosphate crystals have been forming these will then dissolve. Again, vitamin B_6 should be added to the list of supplements.

To summarize, the first priority is to find out whether the urine is acidic or alkaline, and then to start taking the appropriate form of vitamin C.

1 Test urine: if very acid (pH of 5.0 or less) and there is infection, take sodium ascorbate (dosage given below). Taking 1 gram of baking soda between meals and before bedtime (3 grams daily) is also suggested, as this will help to neutralize the acidity in the urine and prevent the high vitamin C intake from irritating the stomach.

2 If the urine is alkaline (pH of above 7.0), take ascorbic acid (dosage given below).

3 In either case take additional vitamin B_6 (pyridoxine).

Dosages

In the case of infection of the bladder, urethra or kidneys it is necessary to achieve what is termed 'saturation' of the tissues with vitamin C. This is done by increasing the dose from 3 grams of the appropriate form of vitamin C (as determined by the acid/alkaline testing) spread throughout the day, by 1 gram per day until the bowels react by the beginnings of diarrhoea. When this occurs, bowel tolerance has been reached, and the dosage will have gone just beyond saturation requirements. In other words, by increasing the dosage daily in this way, the body is tested for its current requirement limit.

Each individual differs in the amounts of vitamin C (and all other nutrients) required. We also need different amounts under varying circumstances: infection and stress are two factors which result in a greater requirement of vitamin C than usual. So one of the easiest ways of asking the body how much vitamin C it requires at any time is to follow the pattern described above, until the body itself indicates it has sufficient (the diarrhoea being the signal). Diarrhoea should cease as soon as the levels of vitamin C being taken are dropped a little. Thus the amount taken on the day previous to the onset of diarrhoea should be resumed and the bowels will normally settle. This level of intake should be maintained until the infection has passed.

However, it is most important not to reduce suddenly the intake once the symptoms have cleared, because a rebound of the infection could occur. The dosage should be restored to normal (1 to 3 grams per day, if prostrate enlargement has been a problem) by reducing the intake by 1 gram per day until this target is reached.

Such a programme of vitamin C supplements is the primary defence measure recommended against bacterial infection of the urinary tract. However, alongside this should go the taking of zinc and essential fatty acids, as described in Chapter 8. No increase in intake of these is necessary, since levels are already adequate for infection, as well as for BPH, as described. (Pollen may be used as a source of EFAs.)

If the cause of recurrent infections of the prostate, urethra and/or bladder is a yeast infection, then the Candida protocol as outlined in Chapter 8 should be undertaken and continued for not less than three months.

Note

In Chapter 8 mention was made of the remarkable benefit of cranberry juice and/or extracts in the case of bladder infections in particular and urinary tract infections in general. These are most effective when there is bacterial infection – stopping adherence of the micro-organism to the mucous membrane which lines the area. Once the bacterial colonies are prevented from sticking to the walls of the bladder or urethra, they are easily 'washed' away by the liquid passing through the region. This approach often gives relief rapidly and should accompany the use of vitamin C treatment, as outlined, but it does *not* deal with the underlying reasons for the infection and of course will have little effect on yeast proliferation.

Catheterization

In some cases where it is impossible to pass water it is necessary for catheterization to be performed to relieve the urine build-up. This, of course, requires expert nursing attention and is not a self-help measure.

Such approaches as hot hip baths or hot towels over the pelvic area can also assist in relief of such a pressure build-up, but should these approaches not be rapidly effective, expert advice should be sought from a doctor.

Once the build-up of urine has been cleared, implementation of the advice given in this and previous chapters will usually be found to achieve remarkably rapid improvement. Full recovery of bladder function, as evidenced by the absence of the various symptoms already described, takes months rather than weeks and requires an ongoing commitment through dietary care.

10
The Key to Prostate Health

What a person eats can have a number of different beneficial effects on the prostate.

First there is what may be termed the detoxification influence which various forms of detoxification patterns of eating can produce. A single period, or repeated periods during which the foods selected are designed with detoxification in mind, would have a cleansing, detoxifying effect on the body as a whole. Methods which could produce this effect include the use of therapeutic fasting: short periods of abstinence from food during which fruit only, juices only, or water only were consumed.

Another influence on the prostate which could derive from the diet is the use of long-term dietary strategies to provide, in food form, the essential nutrients so important for health in general, and prostate health in particular. Such a diet would need to take account of the importance of a reduction in the cholesterol level of the bloodstream. It would also need to focus on bowel health, and so would, of necessity, be a diet high in fibre content. Since this is the type of diet which also protects against diabetes, heart disease and cancer, it can be seen to be a highly desirable dietary pattern.

A further influence of the diet which has to be considered is the fact that attention needs to be focused on those foods and substances which are undesirable and indeed downright dangerous as far as prostate problems are concerned. This should take account of obviously risky foods, such as those with a high fat or high sugar content, as well as foods to which the individual might be sensitive or allergic, since such reactions can produce influences on the urinary tract in general and the prostate in particular.

By taking into account detoxification, nutritional requirements and undesirable – toxic and allergic – influences when trying to construct a 'prostate diet', a plan of action can be produced which largely eliminates from the diet undesirable substances, as well as incorporating into everyday eating those foods which are rich in the nutrients necessary for prostate health.

Into such a pattern it is then possible to build periods of elimination or detoxification. These can be introduced weekly, monthly or at whatever interval is most beneficial, and can last for one to two days or more each as cleansing/detox periods, or for weeks at a time as 'elimination' periods for purposes of identifying food sensitivities, depending upon the needs and general health of the individual.

Detoxification Caution
If anyone is considering undertaking regular detoxification days, then advice should be sought prior to commencing from a qualified naturopathic practitioner, a nutritional counsellor, a clinical ecologist or a medically qualified individual trained in nutritional medicine.

Why Detoxification and Fasting Help to Produce Better Health

Your mind-body defends itself against and copes with invading micro-organisms, toxic materials, changes in temperature, unpleasant situations and a bewildering variety of stresses and strains, of a mechanical (for example, posture), biochemical and emotional nature. For our entire lives we are in a state of adaptation, as this struggle to retain balance – equilibrium – continues.

Your body repairs itself, given the chance – broken bones mend, cuts heal and the vast majority of infections are dealt with efficiently and without symptoms. Even when symptoms appear they are often only evidence of the body doing its self-repair and self-healing work. Fever, inflammation, diarrhoea, vomiting and many skin complaints are all evidence of the immune and other repair systems of the body performing their survival tasks.

Many emotions such as anxiety and depression are only evidence of excessive degrees of perfectly normal emotions. It would be abnormal not to feel anxious in a situation of danger – however, an excessive amount of anxiety is not normal.

In just the same way, allergies are often evidence of an over-reaction on the part of the defence systems of the body to undesirable substances, to which some reaction is perfectly normal.

While physical symptoms are often unpleasant they are often lifesaving – think of the pain of an appendix about to burst; without it, death would arrive silently. Without fever the body could not deal with invading microbes, viruses, parasites, etc. Without inflammatory processes, the repair of damaged tissues could not take place. Without the ability to purge ourselves rapidly of the danger (vomiting, diarrhoea, etc.), poisons could rapidly kill us … and so on.

On a less dramatic scale we can see that a host of stress factors are making demands on our adaptation and repair processes all the time – both emotionally and biochemically, through toxic exposure, the relatively denatured quality of our food and the major emotional stresses of modern life. These multiple and complex demands can ultimately overwhelm our capacity to adapt – especially if they are interacting on a mind-body complex which has inherited imbalances and weaknesses from the start. A gradual decline in health therefore becomes inevitable, often signalled by the onset of what has been called 'vertical ill-health' in which we develop a range of minor symptoms which are not severe enough to send us to bed (horizontal ill-health) and which are seen as 'normal' because so many others have the same problems – ranging from digestive problems to minor skin complaints, recurrent infection, headaches, disturbed sleep, aches and pains, etc.

What's to Be Done about 'the Stress of Life'?

There are only three strategies which can offer a beneficial change to the inevitable decline in health caused by biochemical, mechanical and emotional stressors impacting your defence systems:

a You can try to *remove the causes* (eat better, exercise better, sleep better, relax more, etc.), so reducing the demands being made on the adaptive, repair and defence capabilities of the body.

b You can try to *improve the adaptive, repair and defence capabilities of the body* by methods which enhance immune and repair functions.

c   You can *treat the symptoms* – either in a way which
    causes no new problems (the ideal) or in ways
    which mask symptoms and actually create new
    problems – which is bad medicine.

Examples of this last point are the use of anti-inflammatory drugs for arthritis, painkillers for a headache
and antacid medication for indigestion – all of which
can ease symptoms but do nothing to remove causes,
and as a rule create 'side-effects' and therefore new
problems for the body to deal with.

   In summary we can try to reduce the stress load
and/or improve our ability to handle it, or we can try to
palliate the effects of our handling of the load – well or
badly – or of course we can choose to do nothing and
simply crumble under the onslaught.

Natural Healing Objectives

Unlike the use of medication and many types of surgical
intervention, which *impose* solutions or which make
forced alterations to the situation, natural healing methods start by respecting the self-healing (homoeostatic)
potentials of the body.

   This is sometimes referred to as *vis medicatrix
naturae* or the 'healing power of nature'. In some old
texts it is called 'awakening the physician within',
and in more scientific terminology as 'enhancing
homoeostasis'.

Whatever words are used to describe such methods, they appear to work by allowing space, giving a healing opportunity and doing the opposite of forcing a solution, which might offer only short-term benefits.

Fasting sits at the centre of such approaches, along with relaxation and meditation methods, the use of relaxing hydrotherapy methods, the use of non-specific bodywork ('wellness massage' and aromatherapy relaxation methods, for example) and employment of techniques which have a balancing, harmonizing, normalizing influence – including some herbal and acupuncture methods.

None of these methods, in itself, is 'curative', but all allow the body's healing potential to operate more efficiently because they offer the essential time, space and reduced demands which encourage normalization and recovery, irrespective of whatever is wrong.

This is not to say that such methods can produce absolute remedies in all cases, since in many instances the disease process will have created so much change, so much damage, that the best that can be hoped for is that matters do not get worse, or that there is a marginal improvement. This is nevertheless an infinitely better outcome than a steady decline into ever more ill-health.

Natural healing approaches in general, and fasting in particular, can produce spectacularly beneficial results – a return to well-being, to vital, energetic, clear-headed, bright-eyed, clean-skinned, normal-function wellness.

Trevor Salloum, ND, a famous American naturopath, describes the benefits of fasting:

> ... decreased weight, clearer skin, increased elimination, tissue repair, decreased pain and inflammation, increased concentration, relaxation, plus spare time and savings in the cost of food. Perhaps the greatest benefit is the satisfaction that you are taking a major role in improving your health.

Detox

To restore health in cases of chronic health complaints, regular periods of inner cleansing are often necessary. One day per week at least should be set aside for a 'raw food day'; at least once a month this should be turned into a fast day (or better still, a 48-hour fast).

- On raw food days, only fruits, nuts and salads may be eaten as desired, but nothing cooked.
- On fast days, only liquids are consumed. It is important that at least 2 litres (4 pints) of liquid be consumed on such days. This should be spring water or diluted fruit juice (e.g. 50 per cent apple juice/50 per cent water). It is not necessary to stay in bed on fast days, but activity should be confined

to gentle walks and a fair amount of time allowed for rest.

- On fast days the intake of supplements should be stopped, apart from *acidophilus* powder which should be continued at the normal rate.

Monodiets

If you find fasting on liquids only too difficult, then eat one form of fruit only for the two-day fast.

Grapes are an ideal choice and may be eaten, together with consumption of natural grape juice, to form a modified fast with great benefit. The one-day fast involves a 36-hour period, by starting on the evening prior to the fast and ending the morning after the fast. Eat a fruit and salad meal one evening, fast the next day and eat a fruit and yoghurt breakfast the following morning.

Anyone who has previously been following a typical modern diet rich in refined and undesirable foods will probably note, on the first day or so of a fast, some unpleasant symptoms such as furred tongue, slight nausea and a headache. This is evidence of the detoxification process getting under way, with the liver attempting to cleanse the body of the wastes being stirred up by the fasting process. Urine will probably become very dark or cloudy, further evidence of this process. The bowels may not work for a day or so, but this should be of no concern on a short fast as normality will be restored by the body's own efforts. If a longer fast is undertaken – under supervision – and this lack of bowel movement occurs, then an enema may well be suggested, once daily.

A short or modified fast, repeated weekly or every few weeks, will have a marked effect on general health. Skin will clear and appear more elastic, energy will improve, sleep will be deeper, eyesight and all other senses will be keener and a multitude of minor symptoms will disappear. And there should be definite improvements in bladder function and prostate symptoms.

All this takes time – months rather than weeks – and it is not to be anticipated after one or two fast periods only.

There are no dangers from a semi-fast unless cancer or a diabetic state exists, in which case advice needs to be taken first from a qualified practitioner.

Anti-food Sensitivity Elimination Diet

Many people with chronic prostate problems, or with intermittent prostatitis, may have as a contributory influence food sensitivities or intolerances – not true 'allergies'.

There are a several methods which can be used to identify this possibility. One slightly complicated method attempts to exclude from the diet – for a period – the main known food suspects – based on many years of clinical research by allergy specialists. The most prominent allergy-provoking foods are known to be:

- milk and all its by-products such as butter, cheese and yoghurt
- cereal products (grains of all sorts including wheat, barley, rye, oats and millet – but not including rice and buckwheat, which are not grains)
- eggs and all products containing egg
- refined and processed foods and anything containing colourings, flavourings or other additives (preservatives)
- citrus fruits.

One strategy would be to omit all of these from the diet totally for a while, along with any other foods to which the individual has an obvious history of allergy or 'reaction'.

When all of these are cut from the diet this can leave a very limited range of foods to be eaten for several weeks before the gradual reintroduction of excluded foods, one at a time to judge your reaction to them.

This form of elimination, known as an oligoantigenic diet, has been very successful in providing the clues as to what should ultimately be permanently excluded from the diet.

Initially the total exclusion is for just a few weeks, with the gradual reintroduction of foods – one at a time – each new food being assessed for at least four or five days before the next is reintroduced, to see whether symptoms return.

If symptoms improve during the total elimination and if they return when a particular food is eaten again, it is once again eliminated for at least six months to allow the body to become desensitized to it.

If a food is reintroduced and produces symptoms, a period of four or five days is allowed before another food is tested.

If such a strategy is tried it is important to make a careful note of any symptom patterns as the changes are made – both during elimination and especially during reintroduction. Guidance from a health care professional is useful during such test periods.

A Simpler Elimination Diet

The method outlined above is difficult to maintain for many people, so alternative methods have been devised. In one such method you are asked to choose just one of the 'suspicious' food groups mentioned above, and eliminate this from your diet for at least 10 days.

If there is an improvement in your general health condition during the latter part of the 10 days, then reintroduce the food and eat it several times daily for a few days to see if this brings on any return or flare-up of symptoms (bladder urgency, burning, etc.). If so, eliminate the food from your diet.

If there is no change when leaving it out and when reintroducing it, then just continue to eat it as normal. This method is not as efficient as the oligoantigenic diet, but is easier to maintain.

Another way of choosing which foods to test is to focus on any foods which you eat most regularly (daily or more than five times weekly). This could, for example, indicate a number of commonly eaten foods, say bread, and this should be selected for exclusion for 10 to 14 days, during which time symptoms are monitored. If they improve and the food is then reintroduced and symptoms recur, the food is eliminated from the diet for at least six months. If there is a Candida problem (*see Chapters 2 and 8*) and bread is found to be an irritant food, it could be that the yeast in the bread is the problem rather than the wheat, in which case yeast-free forms (e.g. sodà bread) might be acceptable. The only way to find out is to test, and although this simple version of the exclusion diet is easy, it takes far longer to work your way through the various possible irritants than would be the case with one of the other diets outlined above. In the end of course it may be that the symptoms are not aggravated by any particular foods, but in many instances this detective work is useful and very helpful in assisting recovery.

General Dietary Strategy for the Prostate

In order to produce maximum results for the prostate, a general dietary strategy needs to improve bowel health, reduce cholesterol levels in the blood and ensure provision of ample zinc, essential fatty acids and other nutrients through daily food intake.

Bowel function should be regular and unstrained. This calls for a high fibre content in the diet. Fibre comes in various guises. There is the obvious roughage of the cereal variety, found in bran and in the outer casing of unrefined grains such as brown rice, etc. There are also many gentler and more important sources of fibre. These include the gums and mucilages found in fruits, nuts and seeds and in most vegetables, and in all the bean family. These are more effective in removing cholesterol from the blood than the grain-derived fibres (bran, etc.), thus a high fibre intake of the gum/mucilage variety not only achieves the regular movement of the bowels, but also has a profound anti-cholesterol effect.

Cholesterol is a naturally occurring substance which the body makes for itself in abundance. This is important to understand, for far from being an enemy of the body, no single cell of the body can function without cholesterol. It is only when excessive amounts, of the wrong type of cholesterol, are found in the body that alarm bells are sounded. This is not always a simple matter of high levels in the body resulting from a high cholesterol level in the diet. In fact it is known that the cholesterol we eat, in eggs for example, plays but a minimal part in the level found in the body. Rather it is the result of the type of fat we eat and of the amount of sugar consumed. When a high level of saturated fat and sugars are part of the diet, cholesterol levels go up.

Again it is a little more complex than it seems, because there are different types of cholesterol transporters in the blood, called high density, low density and very low density lipoproteins. In simple terms the more harmful types of cholesterol (low density) are now known to increase in the bloodstream, and to do harm from there, when the diet is rich in saturated fat and especially when saturated fat and sugar (whatever the colour of the sugar) are a major element of the diet. Other elements in the diet compound this problem, such as a high coffee intake and alcohol. Fibre is an effective way of tackling this problem, and a diet which is low in sugar, low in saturated fat and high in fibre is an anti-cholesterol diet. This means that it is an anti-prostate cancer diet too.

The major elements required to achieve such a health-inducing diet are whole grains, fresh fruits, nuts and seeds, vegetables and all the pulses. These must form a major part of the everyday eating pattern of the prostate sufferer, or of anyone who wants to avoid such problems. Foods which contain no fibre are the dairy products and meat and fish. These are not, therefore, of any use in a fibre-enhancing programme, although some of them are of extreme importance if adequate protein is to be eaten.

Obviously a choice exists as to whether or not a vegetarian diet is followed. Such a dietary pattern has definite advantages for health, providing it is well structured. There is always the danger on a vegetarian diet that inadequate protein intake will occur, but this can be prevented by taking care as to the combination of such elements as grains and pulses (beans) so that all the amino acids necessary for the body to construct its own first-class protein are provided. A vegetarian diet usually allows for an immediate high fibre intake (unless white flour and white sugar products are being inadvisedly eaten), as well as a reduction in the chances of eating excess saturated fat, which is so much part of a diet containing lots of dairy foods and meat.

If a meat-eating diet is selected, then a reduction in saturated fats has to be considered carefully. Selecting fish and poultry (apart from the skin of chicken) and using only low-fat dairy products goes some way to achieving this. Game is a further choice which lowers the risk of saturated fat being eaten – game, such as rabbit, hare or venison contains an average of only 4 per cent of the body weight as fat. Beef often achieves 30 per cent of body weight as fat. The type of fat is also very different in that the fat from cows, pigs and sheep is mainly saturated, whereas the minimal amount of fat in game is largely unsaturated. Also, do not be misled into thinking that trimming visible fat from meat will achieve the desired reduction, for much fat in pig, sheep or cow meat is not visible.

Fish is a useful source of desirable oils, especially when cold water fish, such as the herring, is eaten.

The essential fatty acids, so necessary to health generally and to the prostate in particular, can be found in many vegetable foods, including seeds such as pumpkin and sunflower, which are also rich in zinc. The green element in vegetables, chlorophyll, is a rich source of vitamins such as A, E and K, as well as essential fatty acids, and so plenty of green vegetables in the diet will add to the balance of these nutrients. Naturally green vegetables also contain (when fresh) a great deal of vitamin C, as well as fibre.

We can see from this review that the type of diet we should aim for should be rich in green vegetables and protein, whether of animal (low saturated fat type) or vegetarian (pulse and grain combinations). It should also incorporate seeds and nuts, which contain other vital elements, and be sparing in dairy produce and the undesirable meats mentioned.

A basic pattern of diet could be as follows:

- *Breakfast:* fresh fruit plus a seed-and-nut mixture (e.g. sunflower, sesame, pumpkin, linseed together with almonds, walnuts, hazelnuts – these can be ground, crushed or chewed up whole as preferred). If chewing is a problem the mixture of seeds, nuts and fruit can be placed into a food processor and reduced to a pulp for easy eating. A seed-and-nut mixture can also be incorporated with oatflakes and moistened with natural low-fat yoghurt or fruit juice. This provides essential fatty acids and zinc, as well as plenty of protein and fibre.

  If still hungry, then wholemeal toast and a no-sugar jam with a cup of herbal tea may be eaten.

- *Mid-morning Snack (if required):* fresh fruit or seeds and nuts (also fresh, for beware of such foods if there is any rancidity – nuts are best cracked personally rather than purchasing them ready-shelled) and/or drink herbal tea, such as Rooibos, camomile, parsley or lemon verbena.

- *Lunch:* a large mixed salad, incorporating as wide a variety of different vegetables as possible. Green leafy vegetables as well as root vegetables (grated fine) can be made into a mixture which provides different tastes, textures and colours, to tempt even the most jaded of appetites. Raw mushrooms, avocado and other unusual ingredients can add to this. Together with the vegetables, have a mixture of nuts and seeds and cottage cheese or other low-fat cheese, as well as a brown rice savoury or a baked potato. If a potato is not eaten, then wholemeal bread can be added. No butter or margarine should be used, but rather a little olive oil on the potato. Dress the salad with an olive oil and lemon juice mixture, or with natural low-fat yoghurt.

Fresh fruit for dessert.

- *Mid-afternoon Snack (if required):* as for the mid-morning snack.
- *Evening Meal:* a cooked protein meal based on either fish, poultry or game, together with a variety of seasonal cooked and raw vegetables. The American habit of always having a side salad is to be recommended.

If a vegetarian choice is made for protein, then any of a wide variety of dishes, suitably described in many cookery books, can be used. This could include grains (rice, wheat, millet, etc.) and pulses (chickpeas, butterbeans, haricot beans, soya beans, lentils, etc.). Also of course there are egg dishes and cheese dishes, although cooked cheese is not recommended. (It is, of course, quite in order to reverse the main meal pattern and to have the cooked meal at midday and the salad in the evening, if this is preferred or more convenient.)

Fresh fruit or yoghurt for dessert.

Foods to Avoid

- Alcohol should be taken very sparingly, if at all. No more than one and a half wineglasses of dry white wine daily is permitted to anyone in good health, if they are hoping to maintain that happy state. If there are prostate problems in evidence, then no alcohol at all should be consumed.

- Coffee, in very small amounts only, is permitted for anyone with prostate problems. This means no more than one cup of filtered coffee daily. Boiled coffee increases cholesterol levels, and instant coffee does not bear thinking about.

- All sugar should be avoided and certainly not consumed as an additive to food, or in the form of sweets, chocolates, pastries, etc.

- Saturated fats should also be considered undesirable. These are found in all animal fats and in most margarines, as well as in all foods which have been fried.

- All foods which have been contaminated by pesticides, or in which artificial colourings, flavourings or other additives have been used should be avoided. Another reason for avoiding animal meats from most farm sources is the inclusion in their diets of hormones which enhance their growth. Some residues of these pass into the body of the person eating the meat, and since these are largely of female hormone origin, they would increase the dangers of prostate enlargement by suppressing testosterone activity.

By following the type of diet outlined here, together with occasional semi-fasts, and ensuring adequate supplies of nutrients as described in previous chapters, the health of the prostate will be restored to as near normal as is possible. In many cases this will mean a return to a completely normal prostate.

It might appear that there are too many elements which all require attention, but concentration on the basic diet (*page 131*), together with the important nutrient supplements discussed (available from most health food stores) will rapidly produce improvement.

If there is an interest in uncovering possible food sensitivities, the exclusion methods already discussed should be tried. Periodic detoxification days also assist in recovery.

The use of the hydrotherapy and prostate massage methods are not essential but offer a degree of extra assistance which can ease the process of recovery which the diet will ensure.

Note

These methods are not designed for use in prostate cancer, although there is little doubt that the basic dietary and supplement approach will improve such a condition, to the extent that this is possible. Surgery in such a case might be advisable, since if there has been no spread of the cancer, excision of the gland can contain the problem. Prevention is by far the better policy; the use of the dietary methods presented will encourage this possibility.

Prostate problems are not inevitable and are mainly curable by self-help measures. This claim is based on countless cases of recovery from benign prostatic hypertrophy and its complications of cystitis, urethritis and prostatitis.

Index

adaptogens 83–4
ageing 83, 86
alanine 33, 78–80, 91
alcohol 17
amino acids 33, 34, 77–80, 91
animal fats 69–72, 76
anti-Candida diet 103
antibiotics 10, 12, 90
arachidonic acid 32
ascorbic acid *see* vitamin C

bacterial prostatitis, chronic 106–7
bathing, hot and cold 42–4, 113
benign prostatic hypertrophy
   (BPH) 1, 8, 16–20
Berberis vulgaris 90, 102
Bifidobacteria bifidum 97–102
biotin 101
bladder:
   infections 11, 19
   inflammation of *see* cystitis
bowel regularity 33–4, 38
BPH *see* benign prostatic
   hypertrophy
Bush, Dr Irving 63

cadmium poisoning 12
cancer, prostate 8–9, 134–5
Candida albicans 11–15, 107
   anti-candida strategy 15, 97–104
caprylic acid 101
carbohydrates, refined 34
catheterization 113
causes 10
Cernilton 81
Chapman's reflexes 57, *58*
Chimaphilia umbellata (pipissewa)
   89, 95
Chinese Medicine (Qigong)
   exercises 55–6
cholesterol 33, 34, 70–1, 115,
   127–8
chronic bacterial prostatitis 106–7
constipation 33–4, 38
Constitutional Hydrotherapy 49–52
Cooper, Dr 73
copper 67, 90
cranberry juice 94, 112
cystitis 92–4

dairy produce 72

detoxification 114, 115–18, 121–2
diet:
  and prostate disease 69–76
  for prostate health 95–7, 114–15,
    127–34
diets:
  anti-Candida 103
  elimination 115–16, 123–6
  monodiets 122–3
  vegetarian 129, 130
dihydrotestosterone (DHT) 17,
  31–2
Donsbach, Dr Kurt 63, 67

Echinacea angustifolia (purple
  coneflower) 89, 90, 94–5, 102
eleutherococcus 83
elimination diets 115–16, 123–6
essential fatty acids (EFAs) 16, 32,
  67, 73–6, 81, 91, 96, 130
Evening Primrose oil 75, 91
examination *see* palpation
exercise 39, 40, 52–6

fasting 116–21
fats, in diet 69–72, 76, 128
fertility problems 2
fibre, in diet 33–4, 72, 96, 115, 127
fish 130
5-alpha reductase 31–2, 84
flaxseed oil 16, 91
food sensitivities 123–6
food sources:
  of EFAs 75–6, 95–6, 130
  of vitamins and minerals 95–6,
    130
  of zinc 63–4, 66–7, 68 par foods,
    to avoid 96–7, 133–4

garlic 102
genital system 5–6
ginseng 34, 82–4, 91
glandular extracts 85–9, 91
glutamic acid 33, 78–80, 91
glycine 33, 78–80, 91

Hart, Dr 73
heavy metal poisoning 11–12
hormone balancing, foods for 96
hot and cold hydrotherapy 42–4,
  113
Hydrastis canadensis (goldenseal)
  90, 102
hydrotherapy 40–52, 113, 134

impotence 2
incidence, of BPH 1, 16
infections 10, 11
intercourse, mechanics of 39–40
intestinal flora, repopulation 102
iron 67
irrigation, in hydrotherapy 40–2

Kakkar, Dr Vijay 44

Lactobacillus acidophilus 97–102
Lactobacillus bulgaricus 97–9
linoleic acid 32, 75
linolenic acid 32
linseed oil 75

massage, of prostate gland 11, 24,
  28–9, 134
masturbation 10
meat 69–71, 129–30
micturition *see* urine
monodiets 122–3

natural healing 119–21
nutritional supplements 77–113

osteopathic massage 56–9

pain 20
palpation (manual rectal
  examination) 9, 24, 25–7, *27*
Pau d'arco tea 102
Pauling, Linus 93
peak stream tests 19
pesticide poisoning 11–12, 17
Pfeiffer, Dr Carl 62–3, 64, 66
phosphorus 65

pollen extracts 34, 81–2, 91
posture 36–9
probiotics 97–102
prolactin 17, 32
prostate cancer 8–9, 134–5
prostate gland *3*
 description 2–4, 25
 enlargement *see* benign prostatic
  hypertrophy
prostate-specific antigens (PSA) 9
prostatitis:
 acute 9–10
 chronic 11
 self-help for 16
 supplements for 92–5
 symptoms of 15–16
protein, in diet 31–2, 34, 77–8, 81
Pygeum Africanus 85, 94

Qigong exercises 55–6
questionnaires:
 on candida 14
 on prostate problems 21–3

raw food days 121
rectal examinations *see* palpation;
 ultrasound
reflex pressure point massage 56–9

Salloum, Trevor 121
scans 9
self-assessment questionnaire 21–3
seminal fluid 6
seminal vesicles *3*, 5–6
Sereno Repens 34, 84–5, 91
sexual activity:
 excessive 10
 orgasms 39–40
sexual difficulties 18
sexual diseases 9–10
steroids 12
stress 118–19
sugar, in diet 71, 72, 76, 128
sulpha drugs 11
supplements *see* nutritional
 supplements
surgery 108–9

symptoms:
 of BPH 18–23
 of prostatitis 15–16

testes 5
testosterone, and BPH 17, 31
Thermo Regulatory Hydrotherapy
 (TRH) 44–9
towels, hot and cold, hydrotherapy
 applications 42–4, 113
trichomonas vaginitis 107

ultrasound 9
urethra 2
urethritis 11, 92–4
urinary tract infections, recurrent
 105–13
urine:
 acute retention 18
 difficulty in passing 2, 15–16, 18
 foul-smelling 15
 frequency 15, 18–19
 peak stream tests 19
 testing 109–10

vegetarian diet 129, 130
vitamin A 65
vitamin BU6u (pyridoxine) 17, 65,
 66, 68, 91
vitamin C 16, 63, 65, 68, 92–4
 high dose supplementation 109–12
vitamin E 75, 91, 96
vitamin F 73

yeast overgrowth 11, 12–15
 anti-candida strategy 15, 97–104
yoga exercises 39, 52–5

zinc 34–5, 60–8
 action of 31–2
 depleted supply 10
 foods for 96
 supplementation 16, 17, 90, 91

zinc orotate 67, 90
zinc picolinate 67, 90